Devotions for Dieters

A 180 DAY GUIDE TO A LIGHTER YOU

DAN R. DICK

BARBOUR
PUBLISHING, INC.
Uhrichsville, Ohio

Devotions
for
Dieters

© MCMXCVIII by Barbour Publishing, Inc.

ISBN 1-55748-953-X

All Scripture quotations are taken from the Authorized King James Version of the Bible.

Published by Barbour Publishing, Inc., P.O. Box 719, Uhrichsville, OH 44683 http://www.barbourbooks.com

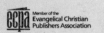

Member of the
Evangelical Christian
Publishers Association

Printed in the United States of America.

DAY 1

? know ye not that your body is the temple of the Holy
t which is in you, which ye have of God, and ye are not
own? 1 CORINTHIANS 6:19

hristians, we believe that God dwells within us. Our bod-
come His home, and it makes sense that we should try to
His surroundings as nice as possible. The temple of God
ael was kept immaculately clean and pure. Only the most
and holy of men were allowed to enter it. It was revered
. The temple was the most holy and special place of all.
we are told that our bodies are the temple of God, it is
option whether or not we will take care of it; it is a duty.
we care for our physical being, we are making God's
le a holy and special place.

Y'S THOUGHT: We diet not only for ourselves, but for God!

DAY 2

ritten, Be ye holy; for I am holy. 1 PETER 1:16

ften we think that holiness is merely a matter of the spirit.
eel that if we read our Bible, pray regularly, and attend
hip, we are being holy. But holiness requires that we ten 1
r physical health as well as our spiritual health. Early
tians realized that they were more alert and better able to
entrate on God when they felt good. Tending to the body
them better at their spiritual pursuits. Dieting may make
ok better, but it will also make us feel better, and it will
le us to pursue God in deeper and more meaningful ways.

Y'S THOUGHT: We please God when we try to be the best
an be!

Day 3

For God hath not called us unto uncleaness, but unto hol[i]
1 Thessalonian[s]

When we try to figure out what it means to be holy, we [think]
of many things that we do which we shouldn't. Our min[ds]
with "thou shalt nots" and we promise ourselves that we [will]
do better. Our minds should not be so filled by the bad t[hings]
we have done; we should focus on the good things we ca[n do.]
Certainly, dieting requires sacrifice, but the benefits inv[olved]
far out weigh the costs. Our focus must be on what we re[ceive]
rather than what we must do without. Dieting is not tu[rning]
from what we shouldn't do. Dieting is doing what God ca[lls us]
to do.

TODAY'S THOUGHT: God will not leave us when we respo[nd to]
His call!

Day 4

For ye are bought with a price: therefore glorify God in [your]
body, and in your spirit, which are God's. 1 Corinthians

Sometimes it is difficult to stick with a diet once it has be[gun.]
If we are dieting for ourselves, we often lose heart, but [if we]
feel we're dieting for someone else, it can be the motiv[ation]
we need to stick with it. Everyday we make promises to [God,]
and those promises we do everything in our power to [keep.]
God calls us to be the best we can be, physically as we[ll as]
spiritually. We should commit our diets to God. If we see [diet-]
ing as a sacrifice we make to God, then we can find a d[eeper]
power to remain committed to our efforts to lose weight[. In]
everything we do honor and glorify God, for that is what [best]
pleases him.

TODAY'S THOUGHT: We are not alone in our attempt to [lose]
weight!

6

Day 5

nfess our sins, he is faithful and just to forgive us our
d to cleanse us from all unrighteousness. 1 JOHN 1:9

e decide for ourselves that being overweight is wrong,
is vital that we put ourselves in God's hands. Though
verweight is not a sin, few people would say it is good.
uld avoid everything that is not good. God will help us
er we turn from things that are bad. Prayer is an impor-
t of our attempts to lose weight. We can trust God to
l our efforts to do what we feel is right. There is no rea-
eel guilty for being overweight, for God forgives us our
ss and offers His own strength as our own. We can start
ts with a clear conscience and an assurance that God is
every step of the way.

s THOUGHT: We have nothing to feel guilty about!

Day 6

nost all things are by the law purged with blood; and
shedding of blood is no remission. HEBREWS 9:22

arn anything at all from being a Christian, we learn that
ings do not come without sacrifice. Jesus had to give
ing He had in order to reunite us with God. If we
to be the best we can be, then we need to accept the fact
re is some sacrifice required. When we learn to sacri-
learn what it means to be Christian. Sacrifice is a good
ne. Sacrifice teaches us what is really important, and it
s be thankful for what we have. When we stop to think
great Christ's sacrifice for us was, it inspires us in our
become better people; people worth dying for!

s THOUGHT: Dieting can draw me closer to being a
e!

DAY 7

But now in Christ Jesus ye who sometimes were far *made nigh by the blood of Christ.* EPHESIAN

A friend of mine who was dangerously overweight la to me once that she was "so fat that God wouldn't even nize me as the person He created." She felt that her problems had driven a wedge between her and God. Ho Nothing that we do ever really separates us from G when we feel badly about ourselves, we feel we are unl even by God. It is important that we see ourselves as go ple. God loves us no matter how we look, but He is de with us when we take pride in who He created us to b will bless our efforts, so we need to draw as close to l possible as we attempt to diet.

TODAY'S THOUGHT: God loves us just as we are.

DAY 8

This is that bread which came down from heaven: not *fathers did eat manna, and are dead: he that eateth* *bread shall live for ever.* JOH

Face it: Dieting wouldn't be so hard if food didn't ta good! Like anything good, we want to get as much of i can. It's easy to place a high value on the food we e there is such a thing as too much of a good thing. G given us many freedoms, but one we should not abuse freedom to consume as much food as we want. No o limit what we eat except ourselves. We need to realize t daily bread supplies what we need, not what we want. sive eating is selfishness, and selfishness is sin. When the urge to overeat, let us turn to God and nourish ourse the true bread that comes from Him—His word.

TODAY'S THOUGHT: God's bread of life is nonfattening!

DAY 9

...dily exercise profiteth little: but godliness is profitable ...ll things, having promise of the life that now is, and of ...hich is to come. 1 TIMOTHY 4:8

... is an old adage that says, "Don't put the cart before the ...' Many people try to lose weight without a specific goal ...d. Often people set a goal that is unrealistic. In our ...ts to become more Christian, we grow a little at a time. ...oesn't expect us to be perfect right away. He knows that ...owth takes time. The same is true of our attempts to lose ...t. We need to take it a little at a time. Crash diets and ...exercise programs are not the way to go. Our Christian ...n should provide us with an example. Let us approach our ...vith patience and take it a small step at a time.

...'S THOUGHT: Dieting is easier if we try to lose weight lit-...little.

DAY 10

...e not conformed to this world: but be ye transformed by ...newing of your mind, that ye may prove what is that ...and acceptable, and perfect, will of God. ROMANS 12:2

...omach is a spoiled brat. When we miss even one meal, it ...up a fuss and makes us feel as though we're going to ...Of course, we're in no danger whatsoever, but once our ...chs get started, it is hard to ignore them. To diet means to ...e in mind over matter. We need to realize that we can get ...a lot less food than we actually eat. We need to renew our ...change our thinking, and decide that we're not going to be ...a slave to our stomachs. We resent it when someone else ...control us. Why should we so easily succumb to our own ...chs? When we refuse to be ruled by anything but the Spirit ...d, then we truly please Him.

...'S THOUGHT: God can liberate us from slavery to the ...ch!

DAY 11

And the peace of God, which passeth all understanding,
keep your hearts and minds through Christ Jesus.

When I get hungry, I get nervous and anxious. I find that
at people and have a very short temper. This is an indicatio
food is more than just a pleasure; it is an addiction. To k
addiction requires restraint and peace. Jesus Christ pro
blessed peace and rest to all who come to Him. It is imp
for us to rely on the gentle comfort of God when we face t
als of dieting. God knows what we are going through, a
rejoices when we turn to Him for peace of mind and hear
not vital that we understand how this peace can come to us
is important is that we truly believe God will grant it.

TODAY'S THOUGHT: In God, there is peace that is greate
the turmoil caused by our dieting!

DAY 12

Draw nigh to God, and he will draw nigh to you. Cleanse
hands, ye sinners; and purify your hearts, ye double min

JAM

Dieting involves a constant struggle between two intense d
the desire to lose weight and the desire to indulge in the foo
love. This is not an easy struggle. We are doubleminded
wants all of His children to learn to be singleminded. On
decide that something is important, we should learn to st
it. That's not easy to do on our own. For that reason
helpful for us to draw close to God. He will listen as we te
troubles. The closer we are to God, the more He can he
through difficult times. If we ask Him to, God will he
become singleminded. He is as anxious as we are to see us
our goal.

TODAY'S THOUGHT: God will keep us on the right track!

Day 13

*t followeth after righteousness and mercy findeth life,
~usness, and honour.*   PROVERBS 21:21

listance runners train themselves to think of the finish
~ey visualize it just ahead. They say this keeps them from
g to give up somewhere along the way. The reward of
g the finish line is worth more than any pain or discom-
the way. Dieters can learn from this. Instead of dwelling
~ hungry we are, or how much we long for rich foods, we
continually think in terms of the rewards that await us at
~. Christians follow Christ with hope of a heavenly re-
Faith means we await something yet to come. Dieting
~ve live in the hope of trimming down and looking fit.

~'s THOUGHT: The reward of our diet is greater than the
~e!

Day 14

*~ righteous Lord loveth righteousness; his countenance
~hold the upright.*   PSALM 11:7

~let self-pity become part of your diet. It's very easy to
~rry for yourself when you diet. First, you feel bad
~e you're overweight. Then you feel bad because of all
~ve to give up. You feel badly because other people don't
~ understand what you're going through. They get to eat
~y please. All of these things can make dieters feel
~ely sorry for themselves. Take heart. God knows what
~going through, and He is delighted that you care so
~about yourself. It is right and good to want to lose
~. Whenever we try to do what we think is right, God
~ts us completely. Replace self-pity with the blessed
~ce that God is on your side.

~'s THOUGHT: Dieting is no reason for self-pity!

DAY 15

*For the eyes of the Lord run to and fro throughout the
earth, to shew himself strong in the behalf of them whos
is perfect toward him. Herein thou has done foolishly: th
from henceforth thou shalt have wars.*   2 CHRONICL

My grandfather always said to me, "You plant your fie
have to harvest it." We made ourselves overweight, a
either have to live with it or work to change it. It is fool
to overindulge, but that doesn't stop us from doing it. A
who is overweight knows well that we have to pay for ov
ishness. True wisdom comes from God. When we deci
enough is enough, that it is time to lose weight, we ca
God will help us, especially through the toughest times.
need do is ask. God is looking for ways to help us, l
always waits until His help is invited. Don't hesitate. Ca
the Lord, and He will hear you.

TODAY'S THOUGHT: If we turn from our foolishness, Go
bless us!

DAY 16

*I am come a light into the world, that whosoever believ
me should not abide in darkness.*   JOHN

When we feel bad about ourselves, we tend to dwell under
cloud of depression. Sometimes we can't think of anythi
but how much weight we've gained and how much we
like to lose. The good news is that darkness always is re
by light. We can get out from under the burden of our weig
can change for the better. Our Lord is a liberator. He f
from anything that oppresses us. Obesity is oppressing, an
is ready and willing to free us. No darkness is too great fo
to dispel. No matter how dark and dismal our physical co
may be, in the light of Christ, we can trim down.

TODAY'S THOUGHT: We always look better in God's ligl
in our own darkness.

Day 17

*ord knoweth the days of the upright: and their inheri-
shall be for ever.*   PSALM 37:18

onestly does know what we suffer through when we try
weight. He sympathizes with us in all our suffering, but
n also see the prize that awaits us. He knows the inheri-
that is to come. Even when we have difficulty keeping
es focused on the goal, we can turn to God, who will
then us by His own strength. He always sees us as what
n potentially be: slim, trim, and healthy. It is important
to try to see ourselves the same way God sees us.
mber, once weight is lost, the struggle is not completely
out we need not ever return to obesity. The fruits of our
, our inheritance, can last forever.

'S THOUGHT: God wants to see us achieve our goal!

Day 18

*ar from me; for them that honour me I will honour, and
hat despise me shall be lightly esteemed.*
                                                1 SAMUEL 2:30

nd of mine played basketball in high school. He did
thing he could to become the best player he could be. He
d with the coach every day. He respected the coach and
erything the coach told him, in order to please him. His
vork paid off. He starred on the team, and when he grad-
, the coach told him he was the finest player he had ever
e privilege of coaching. Are we doing everything we can
ase God by being the best people we can be? When we
ve do God honor, and He will be faithful to honor us in
. If we ignore our bodies, the gift that God gave us, then
ow contempt for God, and He will lose respect for us.

'S THOUGHT: Today I will do everything I can to please

DAY 19

Because Christ also suffered for us, leaving us an ex
that ye should follow his steps. . .Who his own self ba
sins in his own body on the tree, that we, being dead t
should live unto righteousness.   1 PETER 2:

It is good for us to remember, as we sit feeling sorry fo
selves because we may not indulge in tasty pleasures, th
sacrifice is not really so great when we compare it to the
sacrifices Christ made. What we are doing is indeed a
fice, but for self rather than for others. Christ sacrificed
in order that we might enjoy life to the fullest. Let us
from the sacrifice of Christ and remember that He has gi
the power to overcome any temptation that might p
itself.

TODAY'S THOUGHT: Christ has conquered temptation an
be with me!

DAY 20

If thou shalt confess with thy mouth the Lord Jesus, and
believe in thine heart that God hath raised him from the
thou shalt be saved.   ROMAN:

Talk to Jesus. Seriously, He is waiting to listen to you an
you in your struggle to lose weight. Sometimes we w
with the urge to cheat on our diets until we are emo
wrecks. This happens most often when we are alone, w
one to talk to. Don't forget, Christ is always with you, a
is as close as prayer. Tell Him how difficult it is. Let Him
your struggle, and He will indeed comfort you. There is
a time in our lives when Jesus is not interested in every
that is happening to us. Call upon Him, confess Him as
and you will be saved!

TODAY'S THOUGHT: Jesus is as close as a prayer!

DAY 21

...are washed, but ye are sanctified, but ye are justified in ...me of the Lord Jesus, and by the Spirit of our God.

1 CORINTHIANS 6:11

...ny respects, dieting is like a washing away of fat. What ... joy is there than to step up on the scales and see the ... a few marks to the left of where it was a couple days .... When we lose, we feel cleansed, and the cleansing is ...st physical. Emotionally we begin to feel better about ...ves. Our guilt, our poor self-image, our pain all begin to ...away, too. This is the best washing of all. We are ...ed both inside and out, and we become fitting and holy ...s; righteous dwelling places for the Lord!

...'S THOUGHT: Each pound lost cleanses me physically, ...ally, and mentally.

DAY 22

...fore if any man be in Christ, he is a new creature: old ...are passed away; behold, all things are become new.

2 CORINTHINANS 5:17

...people say that what we look like on the outside has ...g to do with what we're like on the inside. This is true ...egree, but how we see ourselves has very much to do ...vhat we think of ourselves. If we see ourselves as over-...t, we will tend to think less of ourselves. If we see our-... as physically fit and trim, then we will feel better. One ...advantages of leaning on Christ when we diet is that He ...e power to make the old pass away and to bring about a ...erful newness to our lives. No one wants our transforma-...ore than Christ Jesus. He's there to help.

...'S THOUGHT: There's a brand new me on the way!

DAY 23

*The Lord rewarded me according to my righteousness: a‹
ing to the cleanness of my hands hath he recompensed ›*
2 SAMUEL

Don't expect God to make you thin. You have to do the ha‹
for yourself. Do know this, however: God will bless you b›
your wildest hopes if you will put forth your best effort a‹
give up. When we show Him that we really are serious ‹
being better people, He is pleased beyond measure, and F‹
do all kinds of wonderful things to help us along. Wh‹
refuse to give into the temptations, to dirty our hands, the‹
will reward us and lift us up. All He asks is that we give ‹
very best effort. If we do that, we will succeed.

TODAY'S THOUGHT: God is pleased by my best effort t‹
weight.

DAY 24

*Righteousness shall go before him; and shall set us in th‹
of his steps.*
PSALM

Jesus fasted for forty days in the wilderness, and He wa‹
tained by His faith. The devil came to Him and tried to ‹
Him with bread, but He refused to give in. This is a ‹
image for us to remember when we are dieting. Often w‹
we cannot go on when we miss just one meal. Christ pro‹
us that even after missing meals for forty days, there is ‹
source of strength other than food. That source is God, ar‹
strength is available to everyone who will ask for it. I ‹
remember to follow in the steps of Jesus Christ and lean ‹
heavenly Father whenever we feel weak or tempted.

TODAY'S THOUGHT: I am facing nothing that Christ did no‹
before me.

DAY 25

Commit thy works unto the Lord, and thy thoughts shall be established.   PROVERBS 16:3

A woman I know carried a pocket New Testament with her wherever she went. Often I would see her pull it out of her pocketbook and begin reading. One day I asked her why she seemed so intent on her reading whenever I saw her. She said, "I read it whenever I get hungry. I'm trying to control my weight, so whenever I feel a physical hunger, I feed myself spiritually instead. It takes my mind off my hunger and puts it where it should be—on the Lord." What a wonderful lesson. If we will find new ways to include God in our diet, He will turn our thoughts where they need to be!

TODAY'S THOUGHT: There are ways to be fed (spiritually) without getting fat!

DAY 26

Blessed are the pure in heart: for they shall see God.
                                                        MATTHEW 5:8

Once we decide something is wrong (being overweight, for example) then doing that thing is sinful. Some may say, "Well, the Bible doesn't say obesity is a sin." The Bible does tell us that anything we do that makes us less than God created us to be is a sin. To be pure in heart means to try to do everything we know we ought to do. We ought to regard our own bodies with respect. We ought to be an example for others to follow. We ought to do all we can to be all we can. When we stay true to what we know in our hearts is right, then we will be assured of a place with God in His kingdom.

TODAY'S THOUGHT: I will do all I can to be all I am meant to be!

For to be carnally minded is death; but to be spiritually minded is life and peace.   ROMANS 8:6

There is a gruesome children's story about a little girl who ate so much that she could no longer move. Then it began to rain, and she died of drowning. Sometimes we try to use terror tactics to get children to do what they should do and avoid things that are bad for them. By the time we're adults, we have forgotten the lessons we were taught as children. There is nothing of any lasting good to be gained from overeating. We need to turn away from what we know is bad, to something better. We need to take seriously the consequences of gluttony, and turn toward God, who will help us change our ways.

TODAY'S THOUGHT: I must set my mind on more important things than food!

DAY 28

He shall send from heaven, and save me from the reproach of him that would swallow me up. God shall send forth his mercy and his truth.   PSALM 57:3

There are going to be days when we feel we just can't do it. Everywhere we turn, there is another temptation, another chance to blow it. Occasionally, we might even give in, but that's no reason to give up. Part of being human means we won't succeed every time we try something. That's okay. When we find ourselves in situations where we give in, that is when we need to call on God, asking for forgiveness, strength, and determination. God shall send forth His mercy and His truth, and we will be able to pick up from where we left off and do even better the next time.

TODAY'S THOUGHT: Losing one battle doesn't mean I've lost the war!

Day 29

If iniquity be in thine hand, put it far away, and let not wickedness dwell in thy tabernacles. For then shalt thou lift up thy face without spot; yea, thou shalt be steadfast, and shalt not fear.   JOB 11:14, 15

A vegetarian friend of mine went to a party and was handed a plate filled with wonderful appetizers. He selected one, took a bite, and then—to everyone's surprise—he threw the remainder across the room with all his might. He stood with a stunned and bewildered look on his face. The appetizer had been filled with meat, and his immediate reaction was to throw it as far away as possible. I think of that whenever I am tempted to grab something to eat that I shouldn't have. In my mind, I have to throw it far away, acting like it is something terrible, so I won't give in to the temptation.

TODAY'S THOUGHT: I will put far away anything that tempts me this day!

Day 30

God is our refuge and strength, a very present help in trouble.
                                                              PSALM 46:1

My grandmother had a favorite picture that showed Jesus stretching out His hand to Peter while they were walking on he sea. It gave my grandmother great comfort to know that if she ever failed in her faith, Christ would stretch out His loving hand to lift her up. Whenever she dieted, she kept that picture close at hand. When the diet got too hard for her to cope with, she looked at her picture and felt God present with her. When we attempt to sacrifice anything, it is good for us to admit that we will have a hard time doing it on our own. When we stretch forth our hand to God, He will always reach back.

TODAY'S THOUGHT: When my diet gets toughest, God will be closest.

DAY 31

The wicked worketh a deceitful work: but to him that soweth righteousness shall be a sure reward. PROVERBS 11:18

It seems too easy to cheat on a diet. There are so many good things to eat, and it doesn't seem like it could hurt to cheat just a little. The problem is, when we try to convince ourselves that a little cheating is okay, then we never seem to draw the line, and a little cheating becomes a lot of cheating. When we are deceitful with ourselves, we find ourselves in big trouble. It is much better for us to do what we know is right, avoiding the things we know will give us trouble. When we stick to our diets, then we can expect nothing but reward.

TODAY'S THOUGHT: There's no such thing as cheating just a little!

DAY 32

My little children, these things write I unto you, that ye sin not. And if any man sin, we have an advocate with the Father, Jesus Christ the righteous. 1 JOHN 2:1

"I can't win," the woman lamented. "I give in and eat something, and then I feel guilty. When I feel guilty, I eat. The more I eat, the guiltier I feel, and the guiltier I feel, the more I eat!"

Sometimes we feel like failures when we break our diets. We can be swept up in a sense of guilt that makes it nearly impossible for us to stick to our diet. The solution to guilt is forgiveness, and forgiveness comes to us through our advocate, Jesus Christ the righteous. Jesus knows that we sometimes give in, and He loves us just the same. Accept His love, accept His forgiveness, and let go of any guilt you may feel.

TODAY'S THOUGHT: I am not condemned just because I sometimes slip!

DAY 33

And by him all that believe are justified from all things, from which ye could not be justified by the law of Moses.

ACTS 13:39

I knew a man who tried a new diet about every two months or so. He would buy the newest diet book and throw himself into the program wholeheartedly. For a week or so, he would remain faithful, then, when results didn't occur fast enough to suit him, he'd fall away. He would curse the diet plans, saying they were no good, completely ignoring his own responsibility to stick to the plan. A book, a law, or a set of rules won't have any effectiveness unless we remain faithful to it. The desire to succeed won't come from a book; it needs to come from a deeper source. For us, that source is Jesus Christ.

TODAY'S THOUGHT: Christ is better than any diet book!

DAY 34

Now unto him that is able to keep you from falling, and to present you faultless before the presence of his glory with exceeding joy.

JUDE 24

There was a girl by the name of Jennifer who was always getting herself into trouble because she couldn't say no. She had absolutely no resistance to any temptation. Then she met Beth. Beth was able to be a voice of reason and common sense for Jennifer. Jennifer knew that if she was tempted, Beth would get her through. Jesus Christ can be to us what Beth was to Jennifer; He can be our voice of reason. Whenever we feel ourselves being tempted, we need to turn toward Him. He is able to keep us from falling. When we find ourselves too weak to handle a situation, we can rest assured that Jesus is indeed strong enough.

TODAY'S THOUGHT: Jesus can keep me on the right track!

Day 35

Iniquities prevail against me: as for our transgressions, thou shalt purge them away. PSALM 65:3

I remember trying to fly a kite at the beach once. I would run as hard as I could in the sand, and it felt like I wasn't getting anywhere. I couldn't run fast enough to keep the kite aloft. Often dieting feels the same way. The harder we try, the farther we seem from our goal. It really doesn't seem worth all the effort it takes. However, we need to hold on. When I tried to fly my kite, a sudden gust of wind came and took it high into the sky. The Holy Spirit of God comes to us just like a gust of wind, helping us reach our goals and making the result well worth the effort.

TODAY'S THOUGHT: Jesus will give us the extra lift we need to lose weight!

Day 36

Let the wicked forsake his way, and the unrighteous man his thoughts: and let him return unto the Lord, and he will have mercy upon him; and to our God, for he will abundantly pardon. ISAIAH 55:7

He loved fried food: meats, vegetables, fish—anything and everything fried. Now he was stuck. He promised his wife that he wouldn't eat any more fried food, but every time he went into a restaurant, the old smells came to him and made both his mouth and eyes water. Time after time, he gave in and indulged in fried delights. Guiltily, he would admit his transgression to his wife, who would scold him, forgive him, and force him to promise not to fall to the temptation again. Forgiveness is important for us to feel when we fall, but we shouldn't take advantage of it. We must always try our best to keep our promises and not ask forgiveness lightly.

TODAY'S THOUGHT: We need fear no condemnation from God when we fall!

Day 37

There hath no temptation taken you but such as is common to man: but God is faithful, who will not suffer you to be tempted above that ye are able; but will with the temptation also make a way to escape, that ye may be able to bear it.

1 CORINTHIANS 10:13

There are going to be times when we feel like throwing up our hands and saying, "I just can't do it!" Dieting is not easy. Don't let anyone tell you that it is. We wouldn't need to diet if we could eat what we wanted when we wanted it. But know this: God will make sure we can hang on, if we include Him in our diet attempts. He knows how hard it is and how much we struggle. No matter how tempted we might be, He will help us escape it.

TODAY'S THOUGHT: There is a way to beat every temptation!

Day 38

But I have prayed for thee, that thy faith fail not: and when thou art converted, strengthen thy brethren. LUKE 22:32

Everyone always wanted Brad on their team. He was tall and very athletic, and every team he ever played for seemed to win. There was also something about Brad that brought out the best in everyone else.

It's good to have someone on our side who can swing the odds in our favor. Jesus Christ is just that someone. He promised His disciples that He would pray for them and they could not fail in their endeavors. He prays for us, too. Jesus is always on our side, and that makes us unbeatable. As we attempt to lose weight, it is vital that we include Jesus in our plans.

TODAY'S THOUGHT: With Jesus on my side, temptation doesn't stand a chance!

Day 39

Submit yourselves therefore to God. Resist the devil, and he will flee from you.
                                                    JAMES 4:7

The earliest days of a diet are the hardest. There are times when it just seems impossible to resist the wonderful treats that appear everywhere. But resist we must. The reward comes to us when we realize that with each victory over an individual temptation, it becomes all the easier to resist in the future. The largest part of the ballet is to realize that we really can do it. The Scriptures promise us that when we resist temptation (the devil), it will flee from us, and it will trouble us no more. God never makes a promise that He won't keep. The battle's been won.

TODAY'S THOUGHT: There is no temptation I cannot resist!

Day 40

For in that he himself hath suffered being tempted, he is able to succor them that are tempted.   HEBREWS 2:18

When we get particularly low during our dieting times, we feel so alone and alienated. People pat us on the back and tell us they know how we feel, but we know they really don't. There are times we feel certain that no one knows how we feel. Rest assured, though, that Jesus knows how hard it is, and He wants to comfort us, especially when the going gets the toughest. Turn to Him, and He will give you comfort and strength in the darkest times. He's been there before us, and He is willing to walk our path with us. Welcome Him in, and He will grant you comfort.

TODAY'S THOUGHT: No matter how lonely I might feel, Jesus is right beside me!

DAY 41

He that overcometh shall inherit all things; and I will be his God, and he shall be my son.   REVELATION 21:7

Being thin is a wonderful goal. Regaining health and vigor is also great. Looking and feeling good are important, but both pale in comparison with how good it is to please the Lord by being the best people we can be. When we diet, we not only gain physically, but also spiritually. Resisting temptation tones our spiritual being as well as dieting tones our physical being. When we reach our goal in our diet, we reach a second goal, as well: We do what is pleasing to God. When we are faithful to do the will of the Lord, we can rest assured that we have an eternal home with Him.

TODAY'S THOUGHT: Dieting makes me a spiritual overcomer as well as a physical overcomer!

DAY 42

Be not overcome of evil, but overcome evil with good.
                                                    ROMANS 12:21

Fat is the enemy. We have declared war, and it takes every ounce of strength we have to wage the battle. Yet, it is a battle well worth fighting. We sometimes need to look at fat as an enemy. We need to think of it as evil, in order to stay serious about battling it. If we allow ourselves to believe that it is anything less than evil, we stand in danger of learning to live with it. That can never be. It is an effrontery to the Christian life to allow evil to overcome that which is good. Rather, let us always strive to overcome what is evil with what is good.

TODAY'S THOUGHT: I will not rest until the enemy has been eradicated!

DAY 43

The Lord knoweth how to deliver the godly out of tempta-
tions, and to reserve the unjust unto the day of judgment to
be punished. 2 PETER 2:9

I remember when I proposed to my wife, I wanted to call home
and let everyone know. I called, but the line was busy. I was so
excited that I just sat and kept dialing until I broke through. I
must have called a hundred times before my efforts paid off. I
finally got through because of persistence. Persistence is one
of the most important ingredients of a successful diet. The
Bible tells us often that God is pleased by our persistence, and
He will reward us for it. God will deliver us, if we will keep
trying no matter what happens. Just don't give up!

TODAY'S THOUGHT: No matter what happens, I will keep trying
to lose weight!

DAY 44

Blessed is the man that endureth temptation: for when he is
tried, he shall receive the crown of life, which the Lord hath
promised to them that love him. JAMES 1:12

What a great feeling! Kim had gone to the party dreading all the
comments of her friends. When they found out she was on a
diet, she knew her friends would try everything they could to
get her to eat the scrumptious food that would be available. It
hadn't been as bad as she thought it would be, though. Her
friends had tried to tempt her, but she had resisted. It had been
difficult, but now it felt great to know that she could be strong
when she really needed to be. If she could resist the temptations
of her friends, she could resist anything. For the first time since
she started dieting, Kim began to really believe she could do it.

TODAY'S THOUGHT: The Lord provides special strength for each
new temptation!

Day 45

There is therefore now no condemnation to them which are in Christ Jesus, who walk not after the flesh, but after the Spirit.
ROMANS 8:1

Perhaps the worst part of dieting is the guilt that accompanies the desire to break from the diet at any possible moment. For some, dieting becomes a challenge to see how sneaky a person can become, but inevitably guilt creeps in and spoils everything. Dieting requires a good spirit and a hopeful outlook. We can not expect to maintain a good state of mind when we continually condemn ourselves for our failures. We need to resolve to try harder and then forget our failings. When we can forgive and forget, we stand a much better chance of a successful diet.

TODAY'S THOUGHT: Valentine's candy adds to the flesh; the Word of God is less fattening!

Day 46

And he said unto me, My grace is sufficient for thee: for my strength is made perfect in weakness. Most gladly therefore will I rather glory in my infirmities, that the power of Christ may rest upon me.
2 CORINTHIANS 12:9

The little boy tagged farther and farther behind his parents. As his father turned to tell him to hurry up, the little boy sobbed, "I can't hurry. I'm too tired. Carry me." He stopped where he was and lifted his weary little arms.

During our diets, we often feel just like that little boy. We just can't go on anymore; we just don't have the strength. That's when we need to turn to God. In our weakness he brings us strength. You will be amazed at what great endurance the Lord gives to those who stretch out their arms to Him.

TODAY'S THOUGHT: The Lord lifts us up from temptation when we reach out to Him.

Day 47

And thine ears shall hear a word behind thee, saying, This is the way, walk ye in it, when ye turn to the right hand, and when ye turn to the left.   ISAIAH 30:21

Diet plans come and go. Weight comes off, weight goes back on. One thing will not change, and that is the loving kindness of the Lord. When the frustration sets in, the Lord is there. When we lose our patience, He will forgive. The Lord is our closest ally and our strongest supporter. We may decide that a particular diet plan isn't for us, or that we need to try something new, but we can never afford to turn away from God. God will help us with whatever plan we choose to follow.

TODAY'S THOUGHT: Any attempt I make to lose weight is incomplete without God!

Day 48

These things I have spoken unto you, that in me ye might have peace. In the world ye shall have tribulation: but be of good cheer; I have overcome the world.   JOHN 16:33

Sometimes we just get tired of dieting. It takes a lot of energy to diet, and without the foods we love, we're sometimes too weak to fight any longer. Our diets become bigger and bigger burdens. If we're not careful, we can lose sight of the fact that our diet won't last forever. All things come to an end if we will only be patient enough to wait. It helps to remember the temptations of Christ; how He triumphed over them, and then, before long, how they ended. Dieting is not punishment, but discipline. Though it can be a tribulation, losing weight carries with it a special joy.

TODAY'S THOUGHT: As the fat fades, so does the tribulation!

DAY 49

And the God of peace shall bruise Satan under your feet shortly.   ROMANS 16:20

I remember going to a cafeteria with my friend once while I was on a diet. I told my friend that I was only going along to keep him company, but that I wouldn't eat anything. Once there, however, I was drawn to a particular piece of German chocolate cake. I debated with myself for the longest time, then finally gave in and went to the counter to buy it. On my way back to my seat, I turned too quickly, and the cake fell from my tray to the floor, where I proceeded to step on it. I always felt that perhaps God was trying to teach me something. The source of my temptation did indeed end up under my feet!

TODAY'S THOUGHT: Food wasted is better than food waisted!

DAY 50

To him that overcometh will I grant to sit with me in my throne, even as I also overcame, and am set down with my Father in his throne.   REVELATION 3:21

The ultimate goal of our Christian walk is to be like Jesus. The ultimate goal of our diet is to be trimmer and more fit. Both goals require great discipline and commitment. Both goals carry valuable rewards with them. It makes sense to combine the goals whenever we can. If we will diet prayerfully, constantly relying on Jesus Christ for comfort and strength, then we will please the Lord and lose weight at the same time. With Christ we become overcomers, and we are promised that we will share in Christ's reward in our heavenly home!

TODAY'S THOUGHT: I can not be beaten, as long as Christ is on my side!

Day 51

Commit thy way unto the Lord; trust also in him; and he shall bring it to pass. PSALM 37:5

Alice Layden was a woman with no self-control. As long as I knew her, she had been terribly overweight. I hadn't seen Alice for over two years when she showed up one day on my front doorstep. She looked fabulous! When I asked how she had finally done it, she said, "I asked God to help me, and I just kept asking Him. Every morning, every noon time, each evening, and anytime I felt hungry, which was almost all the time, I just said a little prayer for God to get me through. He did it! After I thought I'd just about run out of things to try, I found what I should have known all along. God did for me what I was unable to do for myself!"

TODAY'S THOUGHT: The more time spent in prayer, the less time left to eat!

Day 52

It was therefore necessary that the patterns of things in the heavens should be purified with these; but the heavenly things themselves with better sacrifices than these. HEBREWS 9:23

I took a youth group to a play on Good Friday once while I was fasting. All I could think of was how hungry I felt. I was a little cranky, and I found it difficult to concentrate on the play. Suddenly, I looked at the face of the young man who played Christ. His face was contorted with the pain and suffering of our Lord. I looked at a face which truly mirrored everything Jesus had been through, and I was ashamed at myself for the self-pity I had indulged in. When I compared my minor discomforts with the true sufferings of Jesus, I realized I had nothing whatsoever to complain about.

TODAY'S THOUGHT: I will think of what I have, rather than what I have not!

Day 53

Casting all your care upon him; for he careth for you.
1 PETER 5:7

David was driving everyone crazy. He seemed to breeze through his diet while everyone else struggled. At first, everyone assumed he was cheating on his diet, but when he began losing weight faster than everyone else, they gave up on that thought. It was finally discovered that only one thing made David different from the rest of the group: David was a Christian. He began sharing his faith and told the others they could cast all their cares on the Lord and God would help them face all their trials and temptations. The group not only lost weight, they gained faith!

TODAY'S THOUGHT: As we cast our cares on God, He casts His love on us!

Day 54

The name of the Lord is a strong tower: the righteous runneth into it, and is safe.
PROVERBS 18:10

Kate was so thankful that Dennis was willing to spend time with her. Since she started her diet, Kate had tried everything in her power to keep from being alone. When she was alone, she ate. When she was with friends, she didn't feel the need quite as strongly. When she was with friends who understood her, they helped her keep her mind off food. Dennis was one of those understanding friends. He would talk and laugh and make her forget all about eating. He made himself available as much as he could, and Kate was truly grateful. She felt he was a fortress she could run to, where she would be safe from the temptations of food and drink.

TODAY'S THOUGHT: God gives us places of refuge when we tire!

Day 55

Let no man say when he is tempted, I am tempted of God: for God cannot be tempted with evil, neither tempteth he any man.
JAMES 1:13

A woman I knew once told me, "If God wants me thin, He'll make me thin. Besides, He wouldn't have made so many tempting things if He didn't want me to eat them." The poor woman took no personal responsibility for herself, and within a year of our conversation, she was dead. Her heart just couldn't take the strain any more.

Though God will be faithful to help us, He will not do it all Himself. He does not tempt us, nor does He cruelly tease us. He wants only to help us, but we must want to help ourselves.

TODAY'S THOUGHT: God is not the source of temptation, just the solution!

Day 56

A little that a righteous man hath is better than the riches of many wicked.
PSALM 37:16

"I know my limits," Jean said. "If I only keep a little food in the house, then I won't be tempted to eat too much. If I stock up, I just know I'll end up stuffing myself. It's better to just avoid the temptation altogether."

Often it is better to avoid our temptations rather than try to face them head-on. We can not enter into gluttony if we restrict the amount of food we keep on hand. Often our diets are made successful because of the preventive measures we take.

TODAY'S THOUGHT: Knowing our limits helps us limit our wants!

Day 57

For whatsoever is born of God overcometh the world: and this is the victory that overcometh the world, even our faith.

1 John 5:4

The greatest enemy we face as we diet is not food, or the gnawing hunger we endure. No, the greatest enemy we face is the lack of faith we have in ourselves. When the going gets tough, our tendency is to throw up our hands in surrender. That can not be allowed to happen. As faithful people, we are tied to a special power that comes from beyond us. We are recipients of the holy power of God. That same power raised Christ from the dead and enabled Him to overcome every temptation that this world could throw at Him. With that kind of power, how can we fail at anything we do?

Today's thought: To diet means to do it!

Day 58

That ye might walk worthy of the Lord unto all pleasing, being fruitful in every good work, and increasing in the knowledge of God.

Colossians 1:10

Joining the army requires good physical condition and discipline. This is especially true of the army of the Lord. God gave us our bodies, our minds, and our souls. They are tied closely together, and each is to be taken care of as well as we are able. There is no excuse for flabbiness of body, mind, or spirit. It is important that we strive not only to do what is good for our bodies, but also to avoid anything that might be detrimental. As we avoid temptation, we strengthen our wills and make them over in the image of our Lord Jesus Christ's own will.

Today's thought: When I look my best, I look most like Christ!

DAY 59

Cast not away therefore your confidence, which hath great recompense of reward. HEBREWS 10:35

Jeff came out of the store carrying the large package and shaking his head. He really hadn't wanted to buy the radio, but the salesman wouldn't take no for an answer. He had really been persuasive. After a few feeble attempts to resist, Jeff had finally given in. He just wasn't good at fighting off aggressive people. He needed confidence.

We need to be confident that what we do is right. When we lack the confidence we need, we are easy prey for temptation. Confidence is an important part of dieting. When we stand firm on what we have decided to do, then we will succeed.

TODAY'S THOUGHT: Nothing can sway me from my diet, if I don't want it to!

DAY 60

I will instruct thee and teach thee in the way which thou shalt go: I will guide thee with mine eye. PSALM 32:8

My mother cut out all between-meal snacks whenever weight became a problem for my sisters or me. She kept careful watch on us, to make sure our weight didn't get out of control. I resented it when I was young, but I sure appreciate it now. How wonderful it was to know that someone was watching out for me, making sure I didn't give in to fattening temptations. God will do that for us if we let Him. He will twinge our consciences when we do what we should not, and we need to see that as blessing rather than a curse. By heeding the voice within, we can conquer temptation and lose weight.

TODAY'S THOUGHT: God sees every fattening move I make!

DAY 61

And not only so, but we glory in tribulations also: knowing that tribulation worketh patience.   ROMANS 5:3

The growl of his stomach sounded like a ferocious beast. He felt light-headed and nervous. He kept telling himself that he couldn't really be hungry; it was just his imagination. The gnawing hunger would not abate. Before long, he just felt like crying. As much as he wanted to lose weight, he just couldn't face the beast that growled in his midsection. In disgust, he pushed away from his desk and headed out to eat.

A hard part of dieting is showing our stomach who is boss. When our stomachs rule, we lose. Turn to the Lord when weakness sets in. He will see us through.

TODAY'S THOUGHT: I'm not letting my stomach push me around anymore!

DAY 62

And the Lord, he it is that doth go before thee; he will be with thee, he will not fail thee, neither forsake thee: fear not, neither be dismayed.   DEUTERONOMY 31:8

Sylvia was such a support. She really did know what the other women were going through. Not so long ago, Sylvia had weighed well over two hundred pounds. If anyone had earned the right to speak, it was Sylvia. Somehow it made it easier having someone around who was both sympathetic to the struggle and had been successful. Sylvia was indeed a blessing.

It does help to have others around who have been down the road we are walking. These people can be a great source of comfort and courage. Thank God that these examples exist for us to follow. The Lord will not fail us.

TODAY'S THOUGHT: I have no fear of failure, for the Lord is with me!

Day 63

Teaching them to observe all things whatsoever I have commanded you: and, lo, I am with you alway, even unto the end of the world. Amen.   MATTHEW 28:20

A friend of mine fasts regularly, and to my astonishment, he never complains or seems to be the least bit ruffled by the experience. For myself, I find that fasting changes my whole disposition. I asked him his secret once, and he said, "It's no secret, really. All I do is pretend that the empty feeling in my stomach is really the Holy Spirit moving around, making itself comfortable inside. That way, the gnawing isn't unpleasant but it's quite comforting to think that God is so very close." I tried to follow my friend's advice, and it has worked wonders for me. Try it today.

TODAY'S THOUGHT: I will let my hunger turn my mind to God!

Day 64

And call upon me in the day of trouble: I will deliver thee, and thou shalt glorify me.   PSALM 50:15

Jim's watch alarm beeped as the clock struck four. It sounded every hour and every half-hour. I turned to him and asked him what he had set so many alarms for.

"I'm on a diet. Every time my watch goes off, I take a moment to say a prayer to God. It may sound crazy, but it has made this the easiest diet I've ever tried. It calms me down and gets my mind off food for awhile. I feel like I've got a partner, and you know, it's always easier to do something when you don't have to do it alone."

TODAY'S THOUGHT: I can be brave during the tough times, because God is with me!

DAY 65

And this is the confidence that we have in him, that, if we ask anything according to his will, he heareth us.   1 JOHN 5:14

"God just doesn't want me to lose weight!" said Stephanie. "Each time I try, I fail. If God really wants me to lose weight, He'll help me."

Many people feel just like Stephanie. They think God isn't helping them because they aren't successful in their diets. The problem is that they want God to take the weight from them. That simply isn't the way God works. Instead, we need to know that He will work through us to make us strong enough to face the challenges and trials that await us. We take heart in knowing that God will not let us down, and He will work with us all the way.

TODAY'S THOUGHT: God will grant me courage that will not run out!

DAY 66

But the Lord is faithful, who shall stablish you, and keep you from evil.   2 THESSALONIANS 3:3

All her life she had tried to kid herself and say she didn't really have a weight problem. To admit she was fat would have been to admit that she needed to change her habits. She wasn't ready for that. Then her closest and dearest friend had a heart attack. It really scared her and forced her to look at the truth. She was fat, and nothing could change that fact unless she did something about it. It took a lot of courage to face the truth, but it seemed like a lot less courage than facing a possible heart attack. With God's help, she knew she could face the truth and change for the better.

TODAY'S THOUGHT: God makes me fit to fight fat!

DAY 67

Being confident of this very thing, that he which hath begun a good work in you will perform it until the day of Jesus Christ.
PHILIPPIANS 1:6

Confidence. There are days when we feel we don't even know the meaning of the word. It is hard to stay confident when we feel so weak. It is important that we realize where confidence comes from. Our confidence comes from the Lord. It comes from nowhere else. All we need to do is look at the example of our blessed Lord, and we will see that He alone gives the kind of strength necessary to meet every challenge. The things He overcame cause our dieting efforts to pale in comparison. If Christ is truly our Lord and Master, then we will have confidence enough to succeed.

TODAY'S THOUGHT: I am sure to lose weight because of Christ in me!

DAY 68

And it shall come to pass, that before they call, I will answer; and while they are yet speaking, I will hear.   ISAIAH 65:24

When we feel the weakest and most vulnerable is the time to turn to God. God knows what we are up against, even before we call upon Him. There is no one who cares more about how we feel and how we do than God does. He is our staunchest supporter. He also realizes how difficult it is to face our diets alone. He waits for us to call on Him, but He will not force Himself on us until we call. When we do call, He will act quickly to help us, since He already knows what it is we will be asking. Don't hesitate! Call on God when you need Him most.

TODAY'S THOUGHT: I am never out from under God's watchful eye!

DAY 69

Though I walk in the midst of trouble, thou wilt revive me: thou shalt stretch forth thine hand against the wrath of mine enemies, and thy right hand shall save me.   PSALM 138:7

I went through a terrible time when I first started dieting. Every once in awhile, I would get light-headed and my knees would buckle. It was not only embarrassing, but a bit frightening. When I spoke to the doctor about it, he told me it was just my mind playing tricks on me. He said my stomach was "mad at me" for taking away its extra food. I didn't need as much food, but psychologically, I wanted it. I left the doctor and went out to my car to pray. Whenever I felt the light-headedness start to creep in, I asked the Lord to revive me, and He did!

TODAY'S THOUGHT: God is all the pick-me-up I need!

DAY 70

But and if ye suffer for righteousness' sake, happy are ye: and be not afraid of their terror, neither be troubled.
                                                            1 PETER 3:14

If the example of Jesus teaches us anything, it should be that suffering is a noble and good thing when it leads to a better way. Our diets are definitely the source of suffering, but there is great blessing awaiting all who stick with them. God has promised special blessings to those who keep courage in the face of suffering and don't give in. Losing weight not only makes us look and feel better, but it draws us closer to God and His divine plan for us. Our suffering is not in vain. It is all to the glory of the Lord.

TODAY'S THOUGHT: I will fear nothing, as long as Jesus is with me!

DAY 71

And, behold, I am with thee, and will keep thee in all places whither thou goest, and will bring thee again into this land; for I will not leave thee, until I have done that which I have spoken to thee of.   GENESIS 28:15

When I was little, I just hated to be alone. I was afraid of being by myself. When my family got a dog, it made my fear go away. There was never a time when I was alone again. Just having some other presence with me made a huge difference. Now that I'm grown up, I still have a constant companion who will never leave me alone. That companion is God. No matter what I do, I know I am not alone in the endeavor. My diet is no exception. When I feel the most alone, I just rely on the support of the Lord, and He gives me strength beyond measure.

TODAY'S THOUGHT: God helps us to be the best we can be!

DAY 72

The Lord is with you, while ye be with him; and if ye seek him, he will be found of you; but if ye forsake him, he will forsake you.   2 CHRONICLES 15:2

In this day and age, promises are made easily and just as easily broken. We promise ourselves that we are going to lose weight, then we turn around and cheat at every possible chance. For this reason, we ought to include God in our diets. Whereas we might break promises that we make to ourselves, we stand a much better chance of keeping the promises we make to God. When we break promises to ourselves, we have no one to answer to, but when we break our promises to God, He expects us to explain. Promising God that we will lose weight makes dieting much easier.

TODAY'S THOUGHT: I will lose weight for God's sake!

DAY 73

But whoso hearkeneth unto me shall dwell safely, and shall be quiet from fear of evil.   PROVERBS 1:33

Jesus faced many terrible experiences in His lifetime. The Bible tells of many incidents where crowds of people sought to kill our Lord. Whenever the pressures got too great, Jesus withdrew and spent time in prayer. That is an important lesson for us to learn. There will be times when the pressures build up while we try to lose weight. When the pressures get too much for us to handle, we should turn to the Lord in prayer. He will comfort us, strengthen us, and give us the courage we need to face every new day.

TODAY'S THOUGHT: Jesus will take my mind off my diet!

DAY 74

Fear thou not; for I am with thee: be not dismayed; for I am thy God: I will strengthen thee; yea, I will help thee; yea, I will uphold thee with the right hand of my righteousness.
                                        ISAIAH 41:10

Will the diet ever end? That question gets asked an awful lot. What starts out as a good idea soon becomes torture. Giving up seems to be such a good idea. It's at those times that we need the most strength. We need something to pull us through the really tough times. The love of God is just what we need. God will give us strength and courage and will help us fight off the temptation to quit. Call upon the Lord, and He will uphold you, He will strengthen you, He will stay with you, no matter how tough the diet gets.

TODAY'S THOUGHT: If I can make it through the tough times, I can make it through anything!

DAY 75

Therefore we are always confident, knowing that, whilst we are at home in the body, we are absent from the Lord.
                                                2 CORINTHIANS 5:6

David had never been able to stick to a diet. He had tried a number of times, but nothing seemed to help him lose weight. Then he met Jennifer. She was cute, and friendly, and thin. David was suddenly more ashamed of the way he looked than he had ever been before. He began a new diet, and this one worked. David's whole personality changed. He gained a new confidence and strength of will.

What we struggle with at one point becomes easy when we receive the right incentive. With God as our incentive, we can do wonders. Without God, we are helpless. With God, we can do all things.

TODAY'S THOUGHT: I will make sure to keep God close by all day!

DAY 76

For our heart shall rejoice in him, because we have trusted in his holy name.   PSALM 33:21

The Psalms are a wonderful example of what it means to put trust in the Lord. David shared both his trials and his triumphs with his God. In every situation, David turned to God for guidance and support. David was a spiritual giant because he recognized the source of all that he was and could ever hope to be. We can be like David. If we will turn to God for His strength and courage in the face of our trials, He will provide for our every need. When we diet, we can rejoice in the fact that God will honor and bless our trust in Him.

TODAY'S THOUGHT: The diet I keep will bring me joy and fulfillment!

DAY 77

He found him in a desert land, and in the waste howling wilderness; he led him about; he instructed him, he kept him as the apple of his eye. DEUTERONOMY 32:10

It is vital that we remember how pleasing it is to God when we choose to lose weight. No matter how we look or act, God loves us, but just like earthly parents, when we do our best and look our best, we are most pleasing. God is proud of us when we sacrifice and learn self-discipline. He watches our every move, our every struggle, and He loves us. He will be with us continually. Let us follow His teachings and do all in our power to make Him proud of us; not only in our diets, but in every undertaking.

TODAY'S THOUGHT: I am the nonfattening apple of God's eye!

DAY 78

I am not ashamed: for I know whom I have believed, and am persuaded that he is able to keep that which I have committed unto him against that day. 2 TIMOTHY 1:12

"You can't lose weight. You've never stuck with anything in your whole life." Those words haunt me all the time—everytime I slip and eat something I know I shouldn't. I hate it when people think I'm too weak to succeed in my diet. I hate it even more when I prove them right. Still, being ashamed of failing at my diet is often good for me. If I am ashamed enough, then it helps me stick with it the next time. God has helped me a lot to conquer negative shame. I have committed my diet to Him, and He is true to help me keep on track.

TODAY'S THOUGHT: I'll prove to all my skeptical friends that I am capable of losing weight.

DAY 79

What shall we then say to these things? If God be for us, who can be against us?
ROMANS 8:31

Let's not call it our diet; let's call it God's diet. No, that doesn't mean God has to lose the weight. It means that we diet because it's what God wants of us. If it's God's diet, then God will help make sure that it goes well. He will bless those who diet in His name. It may sound silly to diet for God, but, as Christians, we are called to do everything in His name. We live our lives as an offering to do everything in His name. When we live our lives as an offering to God, then we let the whole world know who gives us our strength and courage. If God is for us, then nothing can stand against us.

TODAY'S THOUGHT: Dieting for God is a joy and a comfort!

DAY 80

As for me, I will call upon God; and the Lord shall save me.
PSALM 55:16

We went around the circle, telling about the diet plans we had tried. Most of the people said they had no luck, no matter what they tried. I was the only one who had succeeded in losing a considerable amount of weight. Everyone looked expectantly toward me when my time came. I smiled shyly and said, "The only thing that I did differently from any of you was to pray. I didn't trust any of the diet plans I saw, so I turned to God, instead. You all can try what you want to, but as for me, I'm going to keep putting my faith in God. He's why I'm thin now."

TODAY'S THOUGHT: All else fails; try God!

DAY 81

Let your conversation be without covetousness; and be content with such things as ye have: for he hath said, I will never leave thee, nor forsake thee.　　　　　　　　HEBREWS 13:5

"I hate Sheila," Karen said. "Ever since she lost weight, she's been impossible to be around. She thinks she's so special."

Unfortunately, Karen suffered from a common problem. Sheila hadn't changed. Karen just felt guilty whenever Sheila came around, because she wasn't able to lose weight like Sheila had. Instead of sharing in Sheila's victory, Karen fell victim to jealousy and a bad conscience. Karen needs to understand that Sheila's victory is not her defeat. God will work with each of us where we are. It takes a brave person to celebrate when others succeed where we have not.

TODAY'S THOUGHT: I will rejoice at the example of others who have lost weight!

DAY 82

For the mountains shall depart, and the hills be removed; but my kindness shall not depart from thee, neither shall the covenant of my peace be removed, saith the Lord that hath mercy on thee.　　　　　　　　ISAIAH 54:10

There are times when we feel God has left us to struggle on our own. No matter how we pray, how we plead, it seems no help will come to us. The temptations mount, and our strength and willpower get weaker and weaker. This is where faith comes in. In those times we feel God is absent from us, we must believe that He is still there. God will never leave us, no matter how we may feel. He stays constant for His children. Nothing can move God from our hearts, and we need to know that. God will give us strength in time of need. He will not abandon us, ever.

TODAY'S THOUGHT: I may lose weight, but I can't lose God.

Day 83

What man is he that feareth the Lord? him shall he teach in the way that he shall choose. PSALM 25:12

A group at the church decided to help one another lose weight. A friend of one of the members joined the weight-loss group, even though he wasn't a Christian. After four or five sessions, the young man left the group, saying, "I thought we would help each other not eat. I didn't know you planned to pray and study the Bible. That junk won't help anyone." As it turned out, the group was quite successful. The young man failed because he wouldn't entertain the idea that God could be any help. Those who believe in God trusted in Him, and they were rewarded.

TODAY'S THOUGHT: God is my secret weapon for success!

Day 84

Draw nigh to God, and he will draw nigh to you. Cleanse your hands, ye sinners; and purify your hearts, ye double minded. JAMES 4:8

The cake looked great. Jim waited as long as he could, then, when his wife left the room, he grabbed a small piece. Thinking he would stuff in quickly into his mouth before his wife returned, he turned quickly, the cake fell from his hand. He reacted instinctively and snatched the falling cake. As his wife reentered, he tried to hide his cake-covered hand, but to no avail. He was caught, and there was no way to deny it. We need to stick to our diets and keep our hands clean of the foods we know we should avoid. Draw close to God and away from food. It's the best way.

TODAY'S THOUGHT: If you cheat, you lose everything but weight!

DAY 85

And he said, My presence shall go with thee, and I will give thee rest.   EXODUS 33:14

The most effective diets are those with planned "cheating" in them. Just as the children of Israel set aside a day for fasting from their daily bread, Christian dieters should set aside a day to indulge in the foods they enjoy. This makes the dieter more thankful for the special treats, and makes the diet much more tolerable as well. It gives us something to look forward to, and it erases guilt from the process. We all need rest, and we will find new strength and courage when we break our diet fast occasionally.

TODAY'S THOUGHT: Even dieters deserve a day off.

DAY 86

The eternal God is thy refuge, and underneath are the ever-lasting arms: and he shall thrust out the enemy from before thee: and shall say, Destroy them.   DEUTERONOMY 33:27

It's strange to think of food as "the enemy," but that's the best way to look at it if we want to be effective in our diets. Taking off the pounds is a battle. In every battle we need ammunition. As Christians, our ammunition comes from the Spirit of God that dwells within us all the time. God becomes our fortress; our refuge against the assaults of fattening foods. If we think we can fight the battle alone, we will find it doesn't take long before we tire. At those times we will wish we had someone to take over. Thank the Lord that God is there, and He never tires of fighting alongside His children.

TODAY'S THOUGHT: Dieting makes losers winners!

DAY 87

For the Lord God is a sun and shield: the Lord will give grace and glory: no good thing will he withhold from them that walk uprightly.　　　　　　　　　　　　　　　　PSALM 84:11

I can remember a time when I was on the verge of tears because I was so hungry. I had fasted for almost five straight days, and some friends of mine walked in eating cheeseburgers. The smell assaulted my nose, and the sight of the burgers caused my stomach to clutch and growl. I look back on that incident now and realize that I could not have made it, if it hadn't been for the Lord.

When I think of God as my shield, I think of all the times I feel like giving up because I'm too weak to fight. At those times I'm all the more thankful that I have God to rest upon.

TODAY'S THOUGHT: When my stomach attacks, God will defend me!

DAY 88

If we suffer, we shall also reign with him: if we deny him, he also will deny us.　　　　　　　　　　　　　　　　2 TIMOTHY 2:12

Jesus Christ arose from the dead, glorified and renewed. Before He could ascend to this glory, He had to suffer many things. Much in this life requires sacrifice and suffering before we can attain it. Ask any dieter. The road to thinness is a rugged one. Before we can stand up trimmer and healthier, we must buck up and buckle down. There is very little that is pleasant about dieting, except the end result. Jesus Christ understands what it means to sacrifice better than we ever can. By our sufferings we draw closer to Christ. One day we will reign with Him.

TODAY'S THOUGHT: The power of Christ lifts me above all suffering!

DAY 89

So that we may boldly say, The Lord is my helper, and I will not fear what man shall do unto me.   HEBREWS 13:6

In a prison camp, the people were starved for long periods of time. One man seemed unaffected by the treatment he received. While others complained about how hungry they were, this one man stood by silently. Finally, he was asked why he seem to be doing so well while the others all suffered so. He replied, "I will not let my captors get the better of me. No matter what they do, they will not wear me down. I am the Lord's, and no one else has any power over my life. Men may take away my food, but only God can truly sustain me."

TODAY'S THOUGHT: The need for bread is all in the head!

DAY 90

And who is he that will harm you, if ye be followers of that which is good?   1 PETER 3:13

Watch out! There are a lot of people who would take advantage of us, just because we are vulnerable. When we decide to lose weight, we find ourselves weak and looking for easy answers. Unscrupulous doctors, slick marketing gimmicks, and shyster con artists make promises and products purely for profit. They feed on poor people who want nothing more than the easiest way to take off pounds. Thank goodness we have a source of strength to resist such come-ons. God will protect us from running off after gimmicks and tricks. He is the true answer and the only way to succeed in everything we do.

TODAY'S THOUGHT: No human plan or gimmick comes close to God's plan!

DAY 91

For ye shall go out with joy, and be led forth with peace: the mountains and the hills shall break forth before you into singing, and all the trees of the field shall clap their hands.
ISAIAH 55:12

Our God is a God with a plan for His creation. Everything was created for a reason. God created us in His image, and His plan for us is to live a full, joyful, creative existence. We can best do this by keeping ourselves fit and trim and healthy. God rejoices, as does all His creation, when we live up to the potential He created in each one of us. When we succeed in our dieting attempts, we take a step toward fulfilling our purpose in life, and we go forth in joy and peace which passes any earthly joy or peace. Praise the Lord.

TODAY'S THOUGHT: Thank you, Lord, for bringing me this far!

DAY 92

But let patience have her perfect work, that ye may be perfect and entire, wanting nothing.
JAMES 1:4

Wouldn't it be wonderful if there were a magic wand that we could wave, and suddenly the pounds would melt from our flesh and we would be the perfect weight? I know of no one who would choose the rigors and demands of a diet over a magic wand. Unfortunately, there are no magic wands, and the only way we can lose weight is to set ourselves to the task— body, mind, and spirit. We need to ask God's help, that we might remain committed to the task no matter how long it takes. When we call on the Lord, He will grant us the patience we so badly need.

TODAY'S THOUGHT: The longer the wait, the less the weight!

DAY 93

For ye have need of patience, that, after ye have done the will of God, ye might receive the promise.　　　HEBREWS 10:36

It seemed like forever before any weight came off. Gerri had cut way back on her food intake and exercised daily. It had been frustrating to step up on the scales day after day to find no real change. She stuck with the diet despite her despair, and now four weeks into the program it was paying off. People were beginning to notice the difference in her. What had seemed so painfully slow, one pound every few days, had finally added up, and she was thrilled. Waiting a little while had paid off, waiting a little more didn't seem nearly as hard.

TODAY'S THOUGHT: I can take this diet one day at a time!

DAY 94

To every thing there is a season, and a time to every purpose under the heaven.　　　ECCLESIASTES 3:1

There are times in our lives when a diet may be easier. In times of stress or tragedy, it may be impossible for us to lose weight. Diets take concentration and commitment. Things may come up to cause us to fall away from our diets, but we need to get started again as soon as possible. Just because we fail once doesn't mean we will fail every time. Pray for God's help and guidance. He will be faithful to help us through the tough times and the times we fail. God will make our way easier through His companionship and comfort.

TODAY'S THOUGHT: There is no better time to diet than right now!

Day 95

Rest in the Lord, and wait patiently for him: fret not thyself because of him who prospereth in his way, because of the man who bringeth wicked devices to pass. PSALM 37:7

Is there anything worse than skinny people who act as if dieting were no big deal? It is so difficult to hear others criticize our efforts when they have absolutely no idea what we are going through. However, we need to understand that the comments of those who don't understand us really shouldn't affect us. The Lord loves us as we are, and He truly does understand the struggles we grapple with. He has compassion on His children, and He will deal with those who are cruel or unthinking in their dealings with us. Listen to the Lord, not to others who don't know us nearly as well.

TODAY'S THOUGHT: Beware skinny people with fat mouths!

Day 96

And the peace of God, which passeth all understanding, shall keep your hearts and minds through Christ Jesus. PHILIPPIANS 4:7

Leah was still terribly overweight. She had tried dozens of diets, none of which had made an impact. She attended church regularly, and she prayed continually for God to help her with her problem. She realized that she wasn't ready deep down inside, so she often ignored the voice of her conscience and the comfort of her prayers. Leah lived from day to day asking God's forgiveness and resolving to try harder in the future. She told her friends, "When I'm ready, I know God will be there, and I know He will help me lose all the weight I need to."

TODAY'S THOUGHT: Lord, make me ready to lose weight!

DAY 97

I waited patiently for the Lord; and he inclined unto me, and hard my cry.   PSALM 40:1

Leah was not the kind of woman to just make excuses. When she said that God would help her when she was ready to let Him, she wasn't just copping out. A day came when Leah really needed and wanted to lose weight, and she did it. Though it was hard, Leah stuck to her diet, and she gave most of the credit to God. She had lived for years wishing that she could be thin. Only after trying and failing many times was she able to succeed. Waiting on the Lord can be tiring and defeating. However, no one knows us like God does, and if we can wait, He will always do what is best for us.

TODAY'S THOUGHT: Our best effort will always include God.

DAY 98

I, therefore, the prisoner of the Lord, beseech you that ye walk worthy of the vocation wherewith ye are called, with all lowliness and meekness, with long-suffering, forbearing one another in love.   EPHESIANS 4:1, 2

Temper: It seems that the longer you diet, the shorter it gets. Keeping control of our temper is one of the harder parts of dieting. We feel everyone has some word of advice on what we ought to do differently, that no one really understands what we're going through, and no one appreciates all that we do without. It's no wonder we find ourselves a little short-tempered at times. That's when we need to turn to the source of all patience and peace. If Christ is allowed to rule in our hearts, we will find a new depth of tolerance and forbearance.

TODAY'S THOUGHT: Losing weight is no excuse for losing patience!

DAY 99

For it is God which worketh in you both to will and to do of his good pleasure.   PHILIPPIANS 2:13

Jeff made his living as a night watchman at a large company. He sat for hours at a console that housed a bank of television screens. For his efforts, he pulled a sizable paycheck. Many of Jeff's friends criticized him for getting so much for doing nothing. His reply, "Hey, if they're willing to pay it, why shouldn't I get it?"

Too often people look for ways of getting something for nothing. As God's children, we should always be looking for ways to be the best people we can be, not cutting corners, but committing ourselves to the pursuit of God's pleasure.

TODAY'S THOUGHT: Today I will be the best dieter I can be!

DAY 100

For that which I do I allow not: for what I would, that do I not; but what I hate, that do I.   ROMANS 7:15

The lament of dieters everywhere: "But what I hate, that I do!" Then, after doing what we have vowed not to do, we turn the hate inward, and we are forced to deal with so much guilt. Why does dieting have to be so hard? Why can't we ever seem to have enough willpower to deal with all the temptations? The harder we try, the harder it gets. It's enough to drive a sane person crazy and a saint to sin. Praise God that He understands us so well and is ready to pick us up when we fall and set us back on the proper path. God is patient with us when we most need Him to be.

TODAY'S THOUGHT: I will avoid the things I know I should not do!

DAY 101

Be still, and know that I am God: I will be exalted among the heathen, I will be exalted in the earth.   PSALM 46:10

Whenever food comes into my mind and I have the strongest urges to cheat on my diet, I just close my eyes, clear my head, and try to think of all the wonderful blessings God has given me. I ask God to help me, and then I wait very quietly for Him to answer my humble plea. God has never failed me. In some of the toughest situations, I feel His gentle presence, and my hunger and desire leave me. In the quiet times of our lives God comes the closest, because we do not shove Him aside without other concerns. Call upon God, then wait. He will come.

TODAY'S THOUGHT: If I keep my mouth shut, food can't get in!

DAY 102

And Jesus being full of the Holy Ghost returned from Jordan, and was led by the Spirit into the wilderness, being forty days tempted of the devil. And in those days he did eat nothing: and when they were ended, he afterward hungered.
                                        LUKE 4:1, 2

Forty days without food. The thought boggles the mind. And yet, Jesus was able to do it. Though we are not Jesus, we do have the same source of comfort and strength as Jesus did: the Holy Spirit. If we will concern ourselves with filling up with the Holy Spirit, then we will not have so much time to fill up with other things. Just as Jesus was sustained through the forty days, we also will be sustained by the Spirit of the living, loving god.

TODAY'S THOUGHT: Filling up with the Holy Spirit satisfies, and it isn't fattening!

Day 103

Put on therefore, as the elect of God, holy and beloved, bowels of mercies, kindness, humbleness of mind, meekness, long-suffering. COLOSSIANS 3:12

In centuries past, people went without food in order to break their willful spirits. Certain individuals knew they were too concerned with worldly things, and they wanted to humble themselves, so they went without food. A person who hungers loses conceit and cockiness very quickly. God wants us to have spirit of lowliness and meekness. He wants us to shape our wills to His, and He wants us to be patient in all that we do. Dieting makes us very dependent. We are vulnerable, and we need someone to lean on. Thankfully, we have the Lord to lean on, Who will bear our full weight, and never let us down.

TODAY'S THOUGHT: I'd rather put on patience than put on weight!

Day 104

And the word of the LORD came unto him, saying, Arise, get thee to Zarephath, which belongeth to Zidon, and dwell there: behold, I have commanded a widow woman there to sustain thee. 1 KINGS 17:8, 9

Consider the prophet Elijah. The Lord told him to go to the town of Zarephath, where he was to wait for further guidance from God. Elijah waited there three years before the word came! How many of us would have such patience? Our dieting period often seems long, but in comparison with what so many others have had to go through, the time is really quite short. Committed people have always found a special source of patience and courage to get them through any situation. The source of their remarkable faith is the Lord, who makes all things possible.

TODAY'S THOUGHT: I will make a little last a long, long time!

Day 105

Let not your heart be troubled: ye believe in God, believe also in me.   John 14:1

The days will come when we question whether or not we will ever lose the weight we want to. Frustration can set in, and when it does, it makes us feel like such failures. Jesus' disciples found themselves feeling like failures at times in their lives. It was on those occasions that Jesus offered them the most comfort. Jesus understood human nature perfectly, and He came to let us know everything will work out fine. Turn to Christ when feelings of failure get strong. Our Lord of love and peace will not let us feel badly for long. His love truly conquers all.

TODAY'S THOUGHT: True belief brings real relief!

Day 106

Put off concerning the former conversation the old man, which is corrupt according to the deceitful lusts.
                                                        Ephesians 4:22

Fat people aren't bad people. Sometimes we feel inferior just because we happen to be overweight. It doesn't matter whether we're a few pounds over or a lot of pounds overweight. When we're too heavy, it makes us feel bad. Obesity isn't a sin in itself, but often it is the result of sin. Gluttony, sloth, laziness; these things can lead to obesity, and they are sinful behaviors. When we decide to put off these wrong behaviors, we set ourselves on the path that pleases God. Change takes time, but the rewards are always worth the effort.

TODAY'S THOUGHT: There's more to a new me than just losing weight.

DAY 107

Knowing this, that the trying of your faith worketh patience.
                                                            JAMES 1:3

When you get really serious about losing weight, you have no alternative but to develop patience. There are no safe, quick ways to lose a lot of weight. It takes time. The body takes a long time to build up, and it takes a long time to wear down. However, the person who sticks with her diet will be amazed to find that the longer it's adhered to, the easier it gets. A time comes when the diet is no big deal. In many cases, people find they prefer their diet to their former way of eating. Patience is an elusive trait, but once it is attained, it is its own reward.

TODAY'S THOUGHT: Patience would be a lot easier if it didn't take so long to get.

DAY 108

For our conversation is in heaven; from whence also we look for the Saviour, the Lord Jesus Christ.   PHILIPPIANS 3:20

After Michelle promised Susan she would diet with her, she immediately began to regret it. All Susan did was talk about food. Susan had a one-track mind, and she made dieting so much harder for Michelle. Michelle constantly tried to change the direction of their conversations, but Susan always managed to bring the topic back to food. Finally, Michelle told Susan that if she didn't stop, she would no longer be able to be a diet partner with her. The two worked together and found that with some effort, they could steer clear of caloric conversation.

TODAY'S THOUGHT: Lord, turn my mind away from the pleasures of my tummy!

DAY 109

Better is the end of a thing than the beginning thereof: and the patient in spirit is better than the proud in spirit.

ECCLESIASTES 7:8

It doesn't take a genius to agree that the end of a diet is a lot better than the beginning. Oh, how wonderful it will be to finally reach the goal we set for ourselves, to finish this time of trial, temptation, and struggle! The Lord rejoices when we triumph in the pursuits of our everyday lives. He longs to see us happy and fulfilled. Pray to the Lord that He might bring you to the finish of your weight-loss program. He is faithful to stand beside us, granting the patience we need in all situations so we might finish victorious. Praise the Lord!

TODAY'S THOUGHT: This day means I am one day closer to the end of my diet!

DAY 110

And it shall be said in that day, Lo, this is our God; we have waited for him, and he will save us: this is the LORD; we have waited for him, we will be glad and rejoice in his salvation.

ISAIAH 25:9

Barry was a clock-watcher. Instead of occupying himself in activities that would help the time pass more quickly, Barry chose to do nothing. He waited for things to happen, and as a result, he found himself continually nervous and anxious. Barry was never satisfied with the normal course of events. If we approach our diets with the same attitude as Barry, they will be torture for us. Ask God to help channel our attention to other things. Take control and find ways to get the mind on other things. When we wait patiently, engaged in things that are interesting and enjoyable, then we will find the wait is so much shorter.

TODAY'S THOUGHT: There are a lot of things more interesting than food!

Day 111

See then that ye walk circumspectly, not as fools, but as wise, redeeming the time, because the days are evil.

EPHESIANS 5:15, 16

A friend of mine always said, "If we would only spend time doing what we know we should, there wouldn't be any time left over to do the things we know we shouldn't." Simple truth, but hard truth to follow. When we diet, it is helpful to engage in activities that will prevent us from having the time to eat or even think about food. One person I knew joined a number of volunteer organizations, just so he would be too busy to eat all the time. We need to redeem the time that we spend in fattening endeavors, and turn instead to activities that are pleasing to God.

TODAY'S THOUGHT: The busier I keep myself, the thinner I get!

Day 112

Woe unto you that are full! for ye shall hunger. Woe unto you that laugh now! for ye shall mourn and weep.   LUKE 6:25

As Christians, we need to keep in mind that we live in a world of terrible inequality. While we have the opportunities to overeat and overindulge, many people have no such chances. So many people starve. It is surely humbling to realize that much of our obesity comes from living in a culture where we can have pretty much all we want. The Lord Jesus Christ chastised the people of His day who were filled with the good things of life, because they ignored their brothers and sisters who had nothing. As we diet and feel the hunger in our stomachs, we are more aware of the feelings of our neighbors around the world who do not have enough to eat.

TODAY'S THOUGHT: Make me less, Lord: less body, less selfishness, less ego!

Day 113

Therefore I say unto you, Take no thought for your life, what ye shall eat, or what ye shall drink; nor yet for your body, what ye shall put on. Is not the life more than meat, and the body than raiment?　　　　　MATTHEW 6:25

When I began to diet, I realized how much of my time was spent with something to eat or drink in my hands. Before the diet, I had something in one hand or the other almost all the time. I used to spend a lot of time thinking about where I would eat, what I would eat, and how much I would eat. Food was an idol in my life. How foolish it is to live life like that! There are so many things in life that are more important. Spend time in prayer and contemplation, asking the Lord to open the eyes of your heart to all the wonderful things you have missed for so long.

TODAY'S THOUGHT: I want my life to be much more than food and drink!

Day 114

Stand fast therefore in the liberty wherewith Christ hath made us free, and be not entangled again with the yoke of bondage.　　　　　GALATIANS 5:1

Patience gained during the diet is something well worth holding onto after the diet ends. How many people have lamented that they lost weight only to gain it back again? It is so silly to allow such a thing to happen. We struggle so hard to take weight off, why would we ever let it find a home on us again? Dieting frees us from the imprisonment of a fleshy jail. Once free from that, we should never return. Ask the Lord for strength and determination, so that once we liberate ourselves from fat, we may not be taken prisoner again!

TODAY'S THOUGHT: I will not stand for slavery to flesh and fat!

Day 115

Neither give place to the devil. EPHESIANS 4:27

Satan would have us be much less than we have been created to be. He tempts us to gluttony and greed, then makes us feel weak and unworthy. He tries and tests us a thousand ways, and the harder we try to resist, the harder he works to thwart us. The only way to stand firm against the devil is to enlist the power of the Almighty God. Whereas Satan may have a field day with his human foes, he has no effects against God. When we give in to the temptation to indulge, we are really giving in to the plan of the devil to turn us from God. Follow the Lord at all times, and the devil will flee from you.

TODAY'S THOUGHT: Chocolate cake is nothing but devil's food!

Day 116

For I reckon that the sufferings of this present time are not worthy to be compared with the glory which shall be revealed in us. ROMANS 8:18

Long distance runners say they always keep the finish line in their mind's eye. The goal is the important thing. The runner who loses sight of the finish line is lost. In a like fashion, the dieter who loses sight of a newer, thinner self is lost. Diets are worth every effort we give them, though there are many times when the fact slips from our minds. The apostle Paul found great strength in times of suffering by remembering that those who are faithful receive glory in the age to come. If we will keep our thoughts on the reward to come, our diets will be much easier.

TODAY'S THOUGHT: I can suffer today for a new me tomorrow!

DAY 117

In every thing give thanks: for this is the will of God in Christ Jesus concerning you. 1 THESSALONIANS 5:18

It's easy to be thankful when we have everything we want or need. It's when we're forced to do without that thankfulness becomes difficult. Giving thanks for the opportunity to do without our daily bread is sometimes very, very hard. Yet, God is sure to help us when we need help the most. When we feel weak or hungry or unhappy, he will stand beside us and give us comfort. We're lucky to have God to rely on. Be thankful for the love and care of our Lord. In all things praise Him. When we learn to be thankful in our need, we are all the more thankful in our abundance.

TODAY'S THOUGHT: If it is my heart's desire to be thin, God will help me!

DAY 118

Wait on the LORD: be of good courage, and he shall strengthen thine heart: wait, I say, on the LORD. PSALM 27:14

There will be days when everything seems useless and impossible. The temptation to give up will be almost overwhelming. It is in those times of total desperation that we need to cry out to the Lord. The Lord truly will strengthen the hearts of those who call upon Him. The periods of despair will pass; the temptations will pass. What will never pass away is the loving support of God. He stands beside those who put their trust and faith in Him. Call out to God in the tough times. Rejoice with Him when the times are easy. Wait on the Lord, and He will bless your life!

TODAY'S THOUGHT: As the wait goes on, the weight comes off!

DAY 119

If ye shall ask any thing in my name, I will do it.   JOHN 14:14

A man asked help from his brothers, and they had not time. He turned to his children, and they had too many other things to do. He tried his friends, but they were all away. Feeling lonely and alone, he knelt down and prayed. Why is it that we turn to God only after all our other options are closed? God has promised to give us the desires of our hearts, and yet we seek them in a hundred other places. We need to make God our first choice, not our last. Keep the Lord first in you heart, first in your mind, and first in all you do and say. You'll be amazed what it can do for you!

TODAY'S THOUGHT: A new me is mine for the asking!

DAY 120

And a woman having an issue of blood twelve years, which had spent all her living upon physicians, neither could be healed of any, came behind Him, and touched the border of his garment: and immediately her issue of blood stanched.
LUKE 8:43, 44

How can we seriously feel sorry for ourselves when so many people have so little? Certainly, dieting produces discomfort, but it's very slight. We shouldn't let ourselves get carried away, making our diets a bigger deal than they need to be. However, the good news is, if God can take care of the really big things in life, He will have no trouble helping us through the trial of our diet. God gives good things to those who go out of their way to make Him part of their lives. Reach out to touch the hand of the Lord, and He will reach down to lift us above the struggles we face in life.

TODAY'S THOUGHT: The touch of the Lord makes all things fine!

Day 121

Behold, we count them happy which endure. Ye have heard of the patience of Job, and have seen the end of the Lord; that the Lord is very pitiful, and of tender mercy.   JAMES 5:11

The end may not be in sight yet, but it's there somewhere. Ask the Lord for patience to make it work out. Job was beset by dozens of terrible afflictions, yet he kept his faith and his patience. He is a wonderful example for those of us who are dealing with the ordeal of a long diet. The Lord doesn't want us to suffer, even in small ways. When we diet, we open ourselves to a long, hard road of discomfort and struggle. Having the Lord on our side makes the struggle easier and the discomfort manageable. Job knew that as long as he had his faith, he had everything he needed to get by. The same is true for us today.

TODAY'S THOUGHT: Patience makes the fast pass faster!

Day 122

Jesus said unto him, If thou canst believe, all things are possible to him that believeth.   MARK 9:23

All my friends said they didn't think I could do it. They watched me stuff myself so many times; they didn't think I had any self-control at all. I showed them. I knew in my heart I could make it. Sure, it was tough, but I'm no quitter. When the going got the toughest, it just made me more determined to lose the weight. The key is to believe in yourself. God believes in us, even though we don't always deserve His trust. If God can believe in us, then who are we to do otherwise? Pray for God's assurance, and you will find more than enough faith to make it through.

TODAY'S THOUGHT: God believes in me!

DAY 123

And we know that all things work together for good to them that love God, to them who are the called according to his purpose.
ROMANS 8:28

Ed didn't really know what made him decide to try to take weight off, but now he was glad. His doctor had discovered an irregular heartbeat, and he told Ed to be thankful that he didn't have to carry around so much weight anymore, or his poor heart just wouldn't be able to bear the load. Ed secretly thanked the Lord for helping him out. No matter what had motivated Ed to lose weight, by doing so he had saved his own life. It was ironic, but Ed always knew that God makes all things work out for the best. After this, no one could ever convince him differently!

TODAY'S THOUGHT: My diet may be the best idea God's had all day!

DAY 124

He that chastiseth the heathen, shall not he correct? he that teacheth man knowledge, shall not he know? PSALM 94:10

Jill watched the television program to see the author of a diet plan she wanted to try. She settled in, hoping to be inspired by the man who had helped millions lose weight. When he came one, her heart sank. The man must have weighed three hundred pounds! How could you be inspired by someone who couldn't even practice what he preached? She had really hoped that at long last she had found a winner. Every time Jill put her faith in some new fad, it always seemed to fall apart. Jill guessed her mother was right: The only source worthy of her faith was Christ. Perhaps He really could help where everyone else had failed.

TODAY'S THOUGHT: Following fads is frustrating and foolish!

DAY 125

He that handleth a matter wisely shall find good: and whoso trusteth in the LORD, happy is he.   PROVERBS 16:20

Ben couldn't believe all the people he was talking with. They all wanted to lose weight overnight! None of them seemed to be looking at any practical programs. They had all latched on to crash diets with pills and books and foolish promises of miraculous results. Ben sat down and worked out a practical diet that he could live with, so that once he lost weight (and he realized it would take some time), he could stick with the diet and avoid putting the weight back on. When he said his prayers that night, he put in a special request for some common sense for his friends.

TODAY'S THOUGHT: Trust is a must for weight to abate!

DAY 126

But without faith it is impossible to please him: for he that cometh to God must believe that he is, and that he is a rewarder of them that diligently seek him.   HEBREWS 11:6

Denny looked at the enormous jigsaw puzzle with a gleam in his eye. "This is my puzzle, and I'm going to do it all by myself. Nobody else can touch it!" Denny worked at the puzzle long and hard, but grew frustrated as he couldn't get the pieces to work. Finally, in despair, Denny ran to his father and asked him to come make some of the pieces fit.

We can not afford to enter into our diets with the attitude that we don't need help. Like Denny, we will find that we just can't do it by ourselves. Praise God that He is there for us when we come seeking His help!

TODAY'S THOUGHT: I don't have to face my diet by myself.

DAY 127

That the trial of your faith, being much more precious than of gold that perisheth, though it be tried with fire, might be found unto praise and honour and glory at the appearing of Jesus Christ.
1 PETER 1:7

When the heavy-duty drearies set in, it is easy to question whether you believe in anything at all. Dieting is tedious, taxing, and trying. If there is a God, you may ask, why doesn't He just put us out of our misery? The Lord knows what we need, and He brings us through tough times so we might be made better for it. Just as gold is purified when subjected to intense heat, we are purified by our struggles. When we come through a situation, we are able to look back on it stronger than we were before. Trust the wisdom of the Lord, and He will reward you with faith and love.

TODAY'S THOUGHT: I am made stronger every day that I diet!

DAY 128

For ye are all the children of God by faith in Christ Jesus.
GALATIANS 3:26

Sarah loved chocolate, but when her parents found out she was seriously allergic to it, they made sure she never got any. Sometimes when they were out, she would beg for some chocolate, but her parents never wavered. They allowed her other treats, but they were able to stand firm in their denial of chocolate out of the love they had for their daughter.

Our Lord watches all of us as beloved children. He wants us to have good things, but not things that are harmful to us. Overeating is indeed harmful, so we should not be surprised that God doesn't want us to do it.

TODAY'S THOUGHT: Lord, help me avoid things that could harm me.

DAY 129

And they rose early in the morning, and went forth into the wilderness of Tekoa: and as they went forth, Jehoshaphat stood and said, Hear me, O Judah, and ye inhabitants of Jerusalem: Believe in the LORD your God, so shall ye be established; believe his prophets, so shall ye prosper 2 CHRONICLES 20:20

Too many people fail in their endeavors because they have no backup system. When their own strength fails, they have nothing to fall back on. We Christians have a special advantage in the person of Jesus Christ. When we call out to Him, He is faithful to save us. When we believe in God, He establishes us and helps us attain the desire of our hearts. We need never doubt, as long as the power of the living Lord is on our side.

TODAY'S THOUGHT: All my friends may rely on their own devices, but I will rely on the one who makes all things possible: Jesus Christ the Lord.

DAY 130

Jesus saith unto him, Thomas, because thou hast seen me, thou hast believed: blessed are they that have not seen, and yet have believed. JOHN 20:29

Too many of us suffer from Missouri disease. Missourians are noted for their skepticism, and that is why Missouri is known as the "show me" state. We look for some kind of impressive, spectacular sign. If we don't get it, then we disregard the source. God doesn't work through flashy signs and gimmicks. God works quietly and intimately, and He works His will in His own time. We may not always see the results when we want to, but relax; the Lord is at work, and we need have no fear that He will let us down.

TODAY'S THOUGHT: The Lord is helping me, whether I can sense it or not.

Day 131

And Jesus said unto them, Because of your unbelief: for verily I say unto you, If ye have faith as a grain of mustard seed, ye shall say unto this mountain, Remove hence to yonder place; and it shall remove; and nothing shall be impossible unto you.
MATTHEW 17:20

Too often we miss the point of the mustard seed. We think quantity of faith is the determining factor in getting our hearts' desires. Quantity has nothing to do with it. Jesus used the mustard seed to show that we all have at least that much faith, and if we will learn to employ it, we will see miraculous things happen in our lives. Because of our lives in Christ, nothing is impossible for us, including our diets.

TODAY'S THOUGHT: If I can remove mountains, then I can remove pounds!

Day 132

For whatsoever is born of God overcometh the world: and this is the victory that overcometh the world, even our faith.
1 JOHN 5:4

When Jesus faced the devil in the wilderness, He was weak and hungry. He had fasted long and hard, and He would have given anything to be able to break that fast. Bread is a great temptation to a starving man. Yet, Jesus refused to give in to the temptations of the devil. No matter how enticing Satan was, Jesus was able to resist him. By resisting the devil, Jesus overcame him, and in so doing, He overcame the world and all it could offer Him. We, too, can overcome the world by having faith in the one who has already triumphed. No temptation on earth can bring us down, because we follow the one who overcame the whole world.

TODAY'S THOUGHT: I will turn to Jesus whenever I need a faith lift!

DAY 133

For we are saved by hope: but hope that is seen is not hope: for what a man seeth, why doth he yet hope for? ROMANS 8:24

Gwen stopped by the dress shop every few days to look at the gown she had picked out. Though it was a couple of sizes smaller than she wore, she dreamed of the time she could fit into it. It was a perfect gown. She could visualize in her mind's eye how stunning she would look in it. For the next month, Gwen stuck to a strict diet and made her dream a reality. She lost the two sizes and bought the dress she wanted so badly.

We need our dreams, hopes, and plans to make it through our diets. Hope helps us bolster our faith and makes our dreams come true.

TODAY'S THOUGHT: Hoping helps believing!

DAY 134

That ye be not slothful, but followers of them who through faith and patience inherit the promises. HEBREWS 6:12

Beverly held a support group at the church every Tuesday morning. Bev had been enormous before she began her diet, and to the amazement of the entire congregation, she had lost two hundred pounds. After losing her weight, Beverly had determined to help others in their fights to lose weight. Many people found help in turning to Beverly, because they knew she could sympathize with what they were experiencing. Other people had little use for Bev, because her way of losing weight was too demanding. Being Christian often means taking the hard way, but the hard way always offers us the greatest rewards.

TODAY'S THOUGHT: Help me to benefit from the faith of others!

Day 135

And he said unto her, Daughter, be of good comfort: thy faith hath made thee whole; go in peace. LUKE 8:48

When all is said and done, the determining factor in our diet is going to be our frame of mind. No one loses weight who doubts he can do it. The mind is a tricky thing, and it will tell us time and again that there is no way we can hope to succeed. It will create all kinds of monsters for us to overcome, and defeating them is not easy. Only the person who is mentally and spiritually prepared stands a chance of overcoming. When we truly believe in ourselves and our Lord, then we can go in peace, knowing that nothing on earth can get the better of us.

TODAY'S THOUGHT: God is bigger than any craving my mind and stomach can come up with!

Day 136

And immediately Jesus stretched forth his hand, and caught him, and said unto him, O thou of little faith, wherefore didst thou doubt? MATTHEW 14:31

Peter asked the Lord to allow him to walk on the water. Seeing his Master walking on the waves caused Peter to wish to do likewise. However, once he began his walk, he found himself sinking and afraid. What did the Lord do at this sign of unbelief? Did He allow Peter to sink? Of course not! So long as Jesus is nearby, we need never fear for our lives. Jesus Christ reaches out His hand to us when we get in over our heads. Though He wants us to develop unshakable faith, He is forgiving and loving, and He lifts us up when we are too weak to stand up on our own.

TODAY'S THOUGHT: Thank the Lord that Christ holds me up when I'm most down!

DAY 137

Confess your faults one to another, and pray one for another, that ye may be healed. The effectual fervent prayer of a righteous man availeth much. JAMES 5:16

The group began every week by admitting all their transgressions. Having to admit all the wrongs that were done really helped act as a deterrent during the week. It was embarrassing to tell people about the things you shouldn't have eaten, even though they were all friends. What really made a difference was the period of prayer that ended each session. What a source of strength and courage! The group was the best thing Janet had ever gotten into. Dieting was almost a joy when it was done with such good friends. Sharing the experience helped Janet make her diet a success.

TODAY'S THOUGHT: Confession is good for the soul and for the diet!

DAY 138

For by grace are ye saved through faith; and that not of yourselves: it is the gift of God. EPHESIANS 2:8

Jerry was so confident. He knew he could lose weight if he would only knuckle down and try. But it seemed that no matter how determined he got, something came up to thwart him. Whenever friends tried to help him, he told them to leave him alone; he was going to make it on his own.

How sad that some people try to do everything by themselves. It is good to believe in yourself, but not when that self-belief causes you to be less than you can be. Believe in God. Put your faith there. Whatever you find you cannot do, remember that God can do it.

TODAY'S THOUGHT: Thank God for the gift of determination!

Day 139

For therein is the righteousness of God revealed from faith to faith: as it is written, The just shall live by faith.

ROMANS 1:17

Jean had gone to church for years and had always known she was welcome there. Barbara attended a church across town from Jean's, and she was beginning to think it just wasn't right for her anymore. Both women saw each other at an exercise class that met on Monday mornings. One morning Barbara lamented about her disillusionment with her church, and Jean invited her to come to church with her on Sunday morning. Barbara immediately felt at home in Jean's church, and the two women developed a strong relationship. Faith met faith at an exercise/weight class, and a beautiful friendship was born.

TODAY'S THOUGHT: I will use my diet for the glory of God.

Day 140

He that believeth and is baptized shall be saved; but he that believeth not shall be damned.　　　　MARK 16:16

It is so easy to be tossed back and forth in our commitment to our diets. One day they seem worth the effort, and the next they seem like such a drag. It feels like they will never end, and nothing we do makes the time pass any faster. The sad fact is, it is up to us. If we stick to our diets, we'll lose weight. If we cheat, then we can't expect to lose. Just as the Christian who believes receives the eternal reward, and those who don't believe will have no part in it, dieters who remain faithful reap the reward, while those who lose heart receive nothing.

TODAY'S THOUGHT: In dieting, the biggest winner is the biggest loser!

Day 141

If ye abide in me, and my words abide in you, ye shall ask what ye will, and it shall be done unto you.　　　John 15:7

"I don't really believe in God. I keep asking him for things, and I never get them. I want new clothes, a decent car, and I'm tired of working. I go to church regularly, and I pray all the time. The Bible says that if I ask for anything in God's name I'll get it. I think it's a bunch of hogwash."

Too many people think all they have to do is ask, and God will shower them with wealth and luxuries of life. God does indeed want us to have good things, but He tells us that we must ask for things with a Christlike mind. We need to ask ourselves, "Would Christ ask for this?" Ask in the Spirit of Jesus Christ, and God will bless you richly.

TODAY'S THOUGHT: I need God's help to ask for the right things.

Day 142

Now faith is the substance of things hoped for, the evidence of things not seen.　　　Hebrews 11:1

Jimmy wanted the bicycle so badly he could taste it. His mother and father had told him to save for it, and they would help him buy it. He remembered his father saying, "If it's important enough to you, you'll be surprised how easy it is to save your money." He hoped this was true, because he sure wanted the bike.

If we want to lose weight badly enough, we'll be surprised how easily we can stick to our diets. When the goal is great enough, we find sufficient supplies of faith and determination to overcome any temptation.

TODAY'S THOUGHT: I want to be a substantial person without having a substantial body!

DAY 143

Hast thou faith? have it to thyself before God. Happy is he that condemneth not himself in that thing which he alloweth.

ROMANS 14:22

Face it: You're going to give in a few times along the way. You know it, I know it, and most importantly, God knows it. As human beings, we have to face the fact that there are times we are very weak. Too many people condemn themselves and find it hard to go on. That's nonsense. When we fall down and indulge in a special treat we should not have, we should repent of the transgression but not of the happiness the treat gave us. Those things that fatten us are good, and we like them a lot. There is nothing wrong with liking them, and there is nothing to be ashamed of in falling back now and again.

TODAY'S THOUGHT: If God thinks I'm forgivable, who am I to argue?

DAY 144

But we had the sentence of death in ourselves, that we should not trust in ourselves, but in God which raiseth the dead.

2 CORINTHIANS 1:9

Alice walked ahead of me in the lunch line. As we moved along, Alice would hesitate, reach out her hand, then pull it back. After she had done this a couple of times, I noticed that she had three letters written on the back of her hand: GIW. I asked her what they meant. She looked at me and said, "God Is Watching. I figure if I keep reminding myself of that, it will keep me out of trouble."

When we can not trust ourselves, it is good to know there is someone to trust who will not let us down: Jesus Christ.

TODAY'S THOUGHT: Watch me closely Lord. I'm hungry, and I'm weak.

Day 145

Now the just shall live by faith: but if any man draw back, my soul shall have no pleasure in him. HEBREWS 10:38

Helen lamented that she couldn't lose weight, but she hardly ever tried. Oh, she would spend time with her friends talking about diets, and she would go to exercise class and sit on the side of the gym while her friends exercised, and she would buy diet sodas and TV dinners, but she would also buy coffee cakes and ice cream. The saddest thing about Helen was that she couldn't understand why her friends weren't sympathetic to her. Everyone, including God, will sympathize with us when we are giving it our best efforts. However, if we deal with losing weight like Helen, even God will have little patience with us.

TODAY'S THOUGHT: Only fools think they fool God!

Day 146

Therefore, my beloved brethren, be ye stedfast, unmovable, always abounding in the work of the Lord, forasmuch as ye know that your labour is not in vain in the Lord.
1 CORINTHIANS 15:58

The Lord wants us to develop strong convictions. The best Christians are the ones who are unwavering in their faith. God will help us develop a lot of iron so we might become totally committed to whatever we set our minds to. As dieters, we need that kind of conviction. If we can stand firm in our resolve to lose weight, we can become examples of the power of God to change lives, physically as well as spiritually. When we commit our endeavors to the Lord, we raise them above personal goals and make them a part of our faith walk; a walk we never make alone.

TODAY'S THOUGHT: Let my spirit be immovable, not my body!

DAY 147

Be ye therefore followers of God, as dear children.

EPHESIANS 5:1

As children of loving parents, we always knew they would do what was best for us: loving us, protecting us, providing for us, and teaching us. Our parents wanted us to be happy and fulfilled, and they sacrificed much so we could enjoy life. The Bible reminds us that our heavenly Father loves us even more than any earthly parent every could. We should follow the wisdom of the Lord as children follow the loving guidance of their parents. God will keep us from those things we should not have, if we will only ask Him to. Include God in every aspect of your life, including your diet.

TODAY'S THOUGHT: Let me be a little child of God!

DAY 148

So then faith cometh by hearing, and hearing by the word of God.

ROMANS 10:17

"How do I know that God will help me lose weight?"

The question comes up often, and there is only one response to give:

God will help us in every time of need, and He will never turn us away. That is something we just have to know by faith, and we bolster that faith by listening to the word of God: the Holy Scriptures. God makes wonderful promises to His people, and He is faithful to keep each and every one. He will help us understand His will, if we will only allow Him to do it in His own time and His own way. Listen to the promises of God and receive faith.

TODAY'S THOUGHT: I can't hear God if there's fat between my ears!

DAY 149

For which cause we faint not; but though our outward man perish, yet the inward man is renewed day by day.
                                    2 CORINTHIANS 4:16

It is interesting how we feel so much better about ourselves when we lose weight. As the fleshy part of our being diminishes, the spiritual part of us blossoms. As we decrease our body mass, we find that we unburden hidden parts of our being. We are renewed inside as we take care of the bodies we have been given by God. It is not a matter of being perfect, but of being the best we can possibly be. If we will only keep in mind that we are temples of the most high God, then we will be encouraged to do everything in our power to look and be the best that we are able.

TODAY'S THOUGHT: As there is less of me, there is more of God!

DAY 150

Jesus answered and said unto them, Verily I say unto you, If ye have faith, and doubt not, ye shall not only do this which is done to the fig tree, but also if ye shall say unto this mountain, Be thou removed, and be thou cast into the sea; it shall be done.   MATTHEW 21:21

Most people like to feel they are in control of their lives. When they are manipulated or made to feel helpless, they rebel and fight with everything they can. Funny how many of the same people are people who refuse to be ruled by their passions. They ask themselves, "What would Jesus have me do and be?" rather than leaping into situations without any forethought. Christ should be the only ruler of our lives, and when we turn all power over to Him, miraculous things begin to happen.

TODAY'S THOUGHT: The same power that withers figs can wither fat!

DAY 151

Above all, taking the shield of faith, wherewith ye shall be able to quench all the fiery darts of the wicked.   EPHESIANS 6:16

When we diet, we need protection. We really do. Dieting puts us in a very vulnerable position. We are weakened, frustrated, irritable, guilty, and a hundred other things that stir us up constantly. We need a shield to guard us from the onslaught of so many difficult emotions and feelings. The Lord provides us with the shield we need through faith. Believing in a God who cares for us and stands beside us is a great comfort and a very real help in our times of need. God will not let us struggle alone. He is our refuge, our shield against the worst our diets can do to us.

TODAY'S THOUGHT: Oh, Lord, please protect me from me!

DAY 152

For I say, through the grace given unto me, to every man that is among you, not to think of himself more highly than he ought to think; but to think soberly, according as God hath dealt to every man the measure of faith.   ROMANS 12:3

There were three young men who found they were in need of help from their fathers. The first young man went to his father, but his father told him he didn't deserve any help. The second young man went to his father, but he was told he could have only so much help, then no more. The last young man went to his father, and he was given all the help he needed, and then some. The father let his son know that no matter how much he needed, he could always come to him. Our Father in heaven is like the third father. We need much help in getting through our diets, and we can know through faith that God will always be there to provide us with what we need.

TODAY'S THOUGHT: The more I give up, the more God gives!

DAY 153

For now we see through a glass, darkly; but then face to face: now I know in part; but then shall I know even as also I am known.   1 CORINTHIANS 13:12

One thing would really make dieting easier: knowing what the results are actually going to look like. When we diet, we have to hold on to some image we have created in our own minds. Perhaps it is an image crafted from an old picture, or a memory of what we looked like so many years ago. Still, there is no tangible goal we can point to and say, "That is what I will look like when I lose weight." We have to live in hope of something we want, and hope can be scary. Ask God to help you. He will enable us to believe in what we imagine, even when we can't always see it in reality.

TODAY'S THOUGHT: I'll know better why I'm dieting after I'm done!

DAY 154

Beloved, now are we the sons of God, and it doth not yet appear what we shall be: but we know that, when he shall appear, we shall be like him; for we shall see him as he is. And every man that hath this hope in him purifieth himself, even as he is pure.   1 JOHN 3:2, 3

Sometimes we fool ourselves into believing that to be like Jesus means to act like Him or think like Him or pray like Him, and we ignore that we should try to look like Him, too. We don't know that Jesus was thin, but we can be confident that He was not overweight, because He preached moderation and denounced gluttony. He cared for Himself, and He called others to care for themselves, also. How wonderful it would be to be able to stand face-to-face with our Lord and to mirror Him in both His spiritual and physical perfection!

TODAY'S THOUGHT: When people look at me, I want them to see Jesus!

DAY 155

For thou are my hope, O Lord GOD: thou are my trust from my youth.
                                                              PSALM 71:5

A friend of mine slipped into a well when he was a child, and all he remembers of the experience was praying to God and awaiting rescue. He recounts how he felt no fear, because he knew God would get him out of trouble. He placed his hope in the Lord, and he was not disappointed.

Being overweight can sometimes feel like being in the bottom of a deep, dark well, with no way out. But we do have a way out. The Lord is a lifeline and a Savior indeed. If we will place our trust in Him, He will be faithful to lift us out of the dark places and set us fully in the light.

TODAY'S THOUGHT: Lift me from my well of obesity!

DAY 156

And hope maketh not ashamed; because the love of God is shed abroad in our hearts by the Holy Ghost which is given unto us.
                                                              ROMANS 5:5

There will be those days when we feel we're never going to lose any weight. No matter what we do, the pounds stick with us, and we begin to feel foolish for ever supposing we could lose weight. We find ourselves ashamed for believing that we can lose weight and ashamed at having such defeatist thoughts. It's a very hard position to be in. Luckily, we never really have to feel ashamed of the things we try to do that are good and right. Even though we sometimes lose heart, we still have the love and support of the Lord, who will strengthen us and guide us through His Spirit.

TODAY'S THOUGHT: I'm proud of what I'm trying to do!

DAY 157

Wherefore gird up the loins of your mind, be sober, and hope to the end for the grace that is to be brought unto you at the revelation of Jesus Christ.   1 PETER 1:13

Fighters have to prepare for their bouts in every way possible. They train for a long time, working toward physical perfection. They eat properly, rest regularly, follow the instruction of their trainers closely, and psych themselves up. Psyching entails a preparation of the mind that equals the preparation of the body. Dieters need that kind of mental preparation. As the scripture says, we must "gird up the loins" of our minds. We are fighters against fatness, and the only way we can hope to be victorious is to prepare ourselves completely, day by day, in body, spirit, and mind.

TODAY'S THOUGHT: I'm ready for a good fight against fat!

DAY 158

And it came to pass, when he was in a certain city, behold a man full of leprosy: who seeing Jesus fell on his face, and besought him, saying, Lord, if thou wilt, thou canst make me clean.   LUKE 5:12

Being overweight can sometimes feel like having leprosy. Fatness sets us apart from others and makes us feel different. We feel like outcasts, rejected by our "thin is in" society. Our greatest hope comes to us through the power of the Lord, who is willing to help us in every way possible in our attempts to lose weight. Like the man full of leprosy, all we need to do is stretch out our hands to Jesus, and He will make us clean. We do not have to live as outcasts, but as full members of the glorious family of our Lord, and He is waiting to welcome us.

TODAY'S THOUGHT: Fitness, as well as cleanliness, is next to godliness.

Day 159

And every man that hath this hope in him purifieth himself, even as he is pure.   1 John 3:3

One of the best side effects of dieting is the purging our bodies receive. Interestingly, our bodies function best when we eat less. We don't overload our systems, and therefore, they work better. Our bodies get cleaned out, and we feel better. It is easy to forget that we are helping our bodies operate at peak efficiency, and that our dieting cleans our entire system. Few people would mind feeling great, and God wishes for all of us a healthy, happy life. He created our systems to maintain themselves, but they can only do so if we will respect them and care for them properly.

TODAY'S THOUGHT: My body's in need of a good spring cleaning!

Day 160

And when he was come into the house, the blind men came to him: and Jesus saith unto them, Believe ye that I am able to do this? They said unto him, Yea, Lord.   Matthew 9:28

Doubt is a killer. It kills our enthusiasm, our faith, our hope, our initiative, and our dedication. When we begin to doubt that we can succeed in our diet attempts, we lose the most vital ingredient for success. You have to believe. In Scripture, Jesus often asked people if they believed He could do miracles. When they said yes, fantastic things happened, but when they said no, nothing much happened. We need to say yes to God and believe He will bless all of our attempts to lose weight. With God on our side, there is absolutely no reason for doubt to affect us at all.

TODAY'S THOUGHT: I'll try to believe, so more pounds will leave.

Day 161

And we desire that every one of you do show the same diligence to the full assurance of hope unto the end: That ye be not slothful, but followers of them who through faith and patience inherit the promises. HEBREWS 6:11, 12

Dr. Davidson always had a policy with his patients who tried to lose weight. If he wanted them to lose twenty pounds, he told them they were to lose thirty. If they were to lose fifty pounds, he told them seventy-five. He knew that people would set their minds toward their goal, but that most of them would tire along the way. To counteract that, he always set a goal that was beyond what was actually necessary. Though people did indeed tire before they reached the goal Dr. Davison set, they did not give up before they reached the point they really needed to attain. Sustaining our energy for a diet is hard, but with the hand of God guiding us, we can make it.

TODAY'S THOUGHT: The only thing I will give up is weight!

Day 162

Whom having not seen, ye love; in whom, though now ye see him not, yet believing, ye rejoice with joy unspeakable and full of glory. 1 PETER 1:8

When it's all over, we can hardly belive we struggled so much. The reward of losing weight is so great that it wipes out all the bad memories along the way. We experience such a sense of triumph and joy, accomplishment and goodwill. We feel a power from within that helps us believe that anything is possible to us, if we will only have patience, courage, and commitment. God has made us conquerors, and He empowers us to do those things which we set our minds and hearts to. When we live life in hope of glories to come, and pursue those glories with everything we have, the Lord will reward us and bless us richly.

TODAY'S THOUGHT: I may not see it yet, but a new me is right around the corner!

DAY 164

Behold, the eye of the LORD is upon them that fear him, upon them that hope in his mercy; to deliver their soul from death, and to keep them alive in famine.   PSALM 33:18, 19

Hunger can be a terrible, terrible feeling. It is unbelievable that just being hungry can make us feel so sick and weak, but it does. We need to find ways to train our minds to ignore the pleasings of the stomach. We need to engage in activities that will occupy our minds and absorb us, so we won't think of the food we should not have. In days gone by, people used to carry a copy of the gospels with them, and whenever they felt tempted to do what they knew they should not do, they pulled out the Bible and read Scripture until the desire passed. God is a wonderful diversion to occupy ourselves with when temptations arise.

TODAY'S THOUGHT: I'm not dying of hunger; it just feels that way!

DAY 165

But he answered and said unto them, An evil and adulterous generation seeketh after a sign; and there shall no sign be given to it, but the sign of the prophet Jonas.   MATTHEW 12:39

Everybody wants guarantees. Everyone wants an escape clause: Money back if not completely satisfied. Unfortunately, the world doesn't work that way all the time. Often, there are no guarantees. Sadly, many people approach their faith in Christ in a similar fashion. They don't want to believe unless there are guarantees. They want to have some sign that will remove all doubts. There are signs of God's goodness and glory all around us, but we ignore them all too often. God does not promise us that He will take all obstacles from our lives. Instead, He promises to stay with us and help us learn to conquer them. We need no sign: God is with us, and His love is forever.

TODAY'S THOUGHT: Christ is all the guarantee of success I need!

Day 166

And I heard a great voice out of heaven saying, Behold, the tabernacle of God is with men, and he will dwell with them, and they shall be his people, and God himself shall be with them, and be their God.　　　REVELATION 21:3

Indeed, there is strength in numbers. When we stand alone, we are very vulnerable, and it is easy to give in to trial and temptation. When we stand with others who can relate to our situation, we find a special strength that allows us to cope. Our Lord put us on earth to live together; to draw upon the strength that comes through fellowship. We have fellowship with one another and with God. He is with us, wherever we may be. By His presence, He turns our weakness into strength and helps us hang on through the tough times.

TODAY'S THOUGHT: God makes my hopes reality!

Day 167

But let us, who are of the day, be sober, putting on the breastplate of faith and love; and for an helmet, the hope of salvation.
　　　1 THESSALONIANS 5:8

In battle, the helmet is one of the most important protections. Head wounds can be fatal, and so the helmet must be strong. No soldier would think of entering the fray without proper head protection. Thessalonians says that our Christian helmet is the hope of salvation. Christ gives us that helmet. Through the hope we have in Christ, we are protected and prepared to meet the challenges of our lives. Dieting is just one of those challenges, and without hope of success and completion, we are ill-equipped to meet that challenge. The greater our hope, the better our chance to lose weight.

TODAY'S THOUGHT: Lord, give me a helmet which covers my mouth, too!

DAY 168

...Jesus Christ: by whom also we have access by faith into this grace wherein we stand, and rejoice in hope of the glory of God.   ROMANS 5:1, 2

Some days we just need to stop and congratulate ourselves on how far we've come. Perhaps there aren't a lot of outward signs of our diet yet. Perhaps we aren't even close to where we hope to be. Perhaps we still have a long way to go. That's okay. Sometimes we need to rejoice in the progress we've made in order to have the energy to keep on going. The Lord created in six days, and on the seventh He rested. In every endeavor, especially the difficult ones, we need a break to sit back and enjoy what we've done so far. Even if the beginnings are humble, we can feel good that we are devoted to doing something good for ourselves.

TODAY'S THOUGHT: I'm better than I was yesterday, and I can't wait until tomorrow!

DAY 169

That by two immutable things, in which it was impossible for God to lie, we might have a strong consolation, who have fled for refuge to lay hold upon the hope set before us: which hope we have as an anchor of the soul, both sure and steadfast, and which entereth into that within the veil.   HEBREWS 6:18, 19

When waters get choppy and the foul weather blows in, those who sail know enough to drop anchor so they won't be capsized or dashed onto the rocks. We can learn a lesson from that. As we fight to lose weight, we may find the weather a little foul and the waters a little choppy. Thank God that He is our anchor in all situations of stress and turmoil. If we remember to place our hopes in Him, He will protect us from the temptations and desires that threaten to sink our diets. Call upon the Lord, and He will answer you, and you will be saved.

TODAY'S THOUGHT: God makes me immovable in my determination to lose weight!

DAY 170

*Why are thou cast down, O my soul? and why are thou disqui-
eted within me? hope thou in God: for I shall yet praise him,
who is the health of my countenance, and my God.*

PSALM 42:11

Our society would have us believe that the person who tries to
do something is a failure unless he or she succeeds. Very little
honor is awarded the person who gives it her best shot, but
falls short of the goal. How sad, for it is the person who does
her very best who pleases God the most. When we decide to
diet, and we try to be as faithful to it as we can be, then we are
victors in the eyes of the Lord. We need never grow discouraged when we don't lose weight, as long as we are doing the
best job we can.

TODAY'S THOUGHT: I judge myself harder than God does!

DAY 171

*Watch ye therefore: for ye know not when the master of the
house cometh, at even, or at midnight, or at the cockcrowing,
or in the morning.*

MARK 13:35

Diets need to be taken one day at a time. Each new day means
a new diet. If yesterday's diet didn't work, it doesn't really
matter. Whether we diet tomorrow or not doesn't matter,
either. What does matter is today. Too often we get caught up
thinking about all the things we haven't done or dreaming of
all the things we ought to do, and we have no time to actually
do the things we have set before us right now. God's people
live in the present. They learn from the past and hope for the
future, but they make the most of every single moment of
every day. Live for today and see the miracles begin.

TODAY'S THOUGHT: Today's diet will be a success!

Day 172

When thou passest through the waters, I will be with thee; and through the rivers, they shall not overflow thee: when thou walkest through the fire, thou shalt not be burned; neither shall the flame kindle upon thee.   ISAIAH 43:2

Diets are endurance tests. How long can we hope when we feel as if the end of our trial is nowhere in sight? There will be an end to our diets, even though we often can't see it. It is good to know that God is with us, and He is there to listen to us and share with us throughout our diet. God will be faithful to turn every kind of bad situation to good use. God is the source of our hope. Even when we can't see an end, God will give us the strength and determination we need to succeed. We can not be beaten in our diets as long as we place our hope in God.

TODAY'S THOUGHT: I can always make it through just one more day!

Day 173

Thus saith the LORD; Refrain thy voice from weeping, and thine eyes from tears: for thy work shall be rewarded, saith the LORD; and they shall come again from the land of the enemy. And there is hope in thine end, saith the LORD, that thy children shall come again to their own border.   Jeremiah 31:16, 17

Stephanie looked at the pictures from her wedding day. Had she really ever been that thin? How had the pounds found their way onto her body in such a few short years? She determined that she was going to return to her former figure by the end of the year. As a Christmas present to herself and her family, she was going to be able to wear her wedding dress once again. With a great sense of hope, Stephanie worked toward her goal, and as subtly as the pounds had accumulated, they began to melt away. With the help of the Lord, we can always escape the enemy of fat and return to the land of fitness.

TODAY'S THOUGHT: God helps me beat the fat foe!

DAY 174

Having therefore these promises, dearly beloved, let us cleanse ourselves from all filthiness of the flesh and spirit, perfecting holiness in the fear of God.   2 CORINTHIANS 7:1

Barrie never felt good after stuffing himself. He felt weighted down and slow. He was grumpy and irritable. He usually felt sick. Still, when food was around, he couldn't help himself. Other people would watch him eat, and he could tell they thought it was a disgrace. What could he do? Nobody understood how hard it was for him. He wanted to lose weight and pass by second and third helpings, but he just didn't have the willpower. Too bad Barrie didn't have the support of good Christian friends and a commitment to sacrificing for God. With that kind of support, anyone can hope to lose weight.

TODAY'S THOUGHT: There's no reason for me to face my diet alone!

DAY 175

And the Lord shall help them, and deliver them: he shall deliver them from the wicked, and save them, because they trust in him.   PSALM 37:40

Beth thought the program would never end. It had taken her years to control her weight, and it was still hard to be around scrumptious food for very long without overindulging. All through the evening, heavenly plates of food moved around the room. It was all Beth could do to resist. Whenever the temptation arose, she closed her eyes and quietly prayed to God for strength. It seemed like an eternity, but the evening finally ended, and she had somehow made it through. With a sigh of relief, she said a quick prayer of thanks as she walked to her car.

TODAY'S THOUGHT: When I can't make it, God can!

DAY 176

Wherefore thou art no more a servant, but a son; and if a son, then an heir of God through Christ.   GALATIANS 4:7

Kerry knew God loved her when she was fat, but she felt His love so much more now that she was thin. She knew it had nothing to do with how much God really loved her, but with how much she loved herself. Now, she could look in the mirror without shame blushing her cheeks. Now, she could hold her head up and not worry about what other people thought of her. Once she had been a slave to her body. Now she was free to be everything she wanted to be. She had once believed she would never be free of the weight that burdened her, not only physically, but emotionally, too. God indeed worked wonders!

TODAY'S THOUGHT: With God's help, I will be free from fat.

DAY 177

And the peace of God, which passeth all understanding, shall keep your hearts and minds through Christ Jesus.
                                                        PHILLIPIANS 4:7

Promises. Every diet made promises, and they very rarely came through. Jenny had tried a dozen diets, each time putting her faith in their promises. Quietly, with tears in her eyes, she prayed for God's help. She wanted to lose weight so badly. As she prayed, she felt calm and hopeful. If only she could feel so peaceful when temptation raised its ugly head. Jenny vowed to try turning to God for help in the future instead of turning to more fad diets. Maybe God could do things for her that diet plans couldn't. She didn't really understand it, but she believed it was true.

TODAY'S THOUGHT: If I turn to God, there's always hope!

Day 178

Then shall we know, if we follow on to know the LORD: his going forth is prepared as the morning; and he shall come unto us as the rain, as the latter and former rain unto the earth.

HOSEA 6:3

Carol went to a Christian prayer group with some skepticism. Gladys and Ann had started going, and they had immediately made great strides in their diets. Both women gave all the credit to God, but Carol wasn't convinced. She thought it sounded way too easy. Why would God do something for her that she ought to be able to do for herself? Carol wanted to believe, but she just couldn't quite believe that God would be interested enough in her weight problem to help her out. Too bad for Carol that she never realized how trustworthy the Lord is. If we put our faith in Him, He will be sure to help us.

TODAY'S THOUGHT: No matter is too insignificant to bring to God!

Day 179

For every creature of God is good, and nothing to be refused, if it be received with thanksgiving.   1 TIMOTHY 4:4

Greg tried not to get discouraged, even though he gained back most of the weight he'd lost. This time it would be easier. He'd done it once; he could do it again. The first time had been so hard because he had such a low opinion of himself. His self-image had improved immensely, and he had the confidence he needed to know he could lose weight. Greg knew he was made in God's image, even if that image got hidden a little now and then. Knowing that he was loved made losing weight much easier. Greg was thankful that God loved him so. He could conquer anything, with God's help.

TODAY'S THOUGHT: Good things come to those who believe they will!

Be of good courage, and he shall strengthen your heart, all ye that hope in the LORD.   PSALM 31:24

Gail's wedding day was getting close. She had vowed to lose fifty pounds by the time she got married. She was within ten pounds of her goal, but the last ten pounds were the hardest. She was so worried that she might not make it. She sat alone, looking at the dress, and then she bowed her head to pray. As she asked the Lord for help, she renewed her promise to do everything she could to lose the weight. Suddenly, deep inside, she knew she was going to make it. Everything she hoped for would work out, because the Lord was giving her the strength and courage she needed to succeed.

TODAY'S THOUGHT: When God says it will work out, it works out!